FOOT AND ANKLE
Injection Techniques

ACKNOWLEDGEMENTS

Members of the Northampton and Solihull Podiatric Surgery teams for the DVD.

Trish Munday, audio typist and anatomy model.

Professor Ribbans, Consultant Orthopaedic Surgeon, Northampton General Hospital.

Commissioning Editor: Robert Edwards/Sarena Wolfaard
Development Editor: Nicola Lally
Project Manager: Sukanthi Sukumar and Anne Dickie
Designer: Kirsteen Wright
Illustration Manager: Merlyn Harvey
Illustrator: Cactus

FOOT AND ANKLE
Injection Techniques
A Practical Guide

Stuart Metcalfe FPodA, FCPodS

Ian Reilly FCPodS, DMS

Foreword by

Bill Ribbans PhD, FRCSOrth, FFSEM (UK)
Consultant Trauma and Orthopaedic Surgeon,
Visiting Professor, University of Northampton, UK

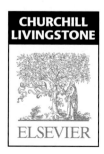

CHURCHILL
LIVINGSTONE

ELSEVIER

Edinburgh   London   New York   Oxford   Philadelphia   St Louis   Sydney   Toronto   2010

CHURCHILL
LIVINGSTONE
ELSEVIER

First published 2010, © Elsevier Limited. All rights reserved.

ISBN 978-0-7020-3107-6

British Library Cataloguing in Publication Data
A catalogue record for this book is available from the British Library

Library of Congress Cataloging in Publication Data
A catalog record for this book is available from the Library of Congress

Notice
Knowledge and best practice in this field are constantly changing. As new research and experience broaden our knowledge, changes in practice, treatment and drug therapy may become necessary or appropriate. Readers are advised to check the most current information provided (i) on procedures featured or (ii) by the manufacturer of each product to be administered, to verify the recommended dose or formula, the method and duration of administration, and contraindications. It is the responsibility of the practitioner, relying on their own experience and knowledge of the patient, to make diagnoses, to determine dosages and the best treatment for each individual patient, and to take all appropriate safety precautions. To the fullest extent of the law, neither the Publisher nor the Authors assumes any liability for any injury and/or damage to persons or property arising out of or related to any use of the material contained in this book.

The Publisher

ELSEVIER your source for books, journals and multimedia in the health sciences

www.elsevierhealth.com

Working together to grow
libraries in developing countries

www.elsevier.com | www.bookaid.org | www.sabre.org

ELSEVIER   BOOK AID International   Sabre Foundation

The Publisher's policy is to use **paper manufactured from sustainable forests**

Printed in China

FOREWORD

Injections around the Foot and Ankle are undertaken principally for three reasons. The first is for diagnostic purposes, the second for therapeutic pain relief, and the final reason to provide anaesthesia as a prelude to surgery.

Clinicians undertaking such an injection must possess a sound knowledge of the area's anatomy and the potential complications following inadvertent damage to adjacent structures. They must be able to assess their patients' suitability for such a procedure and be aware of the increasingly wide range of drugs available. Added to a knowledge of the effectiveness of each drug must be added an understanding of the pharmacology and pharmacokinetics of individual substances. On a practical front, the clinician must be competent in aseptic technique and, with experience, becoming increasingly skilled at providing a successful and as atraumatic injection as possible.

Armed with this theoretical and practical knowledge, clinicians will be able to have confidence in taking the right decisions for their patients and counsel them with assurance prior to the procedure.

The authors have gone to enormous trouble with this book to assemble all of the information required for a clinician in this important and commonly required area of foot and ankle care and present it in a readable and enjoyable format beautifully illustrated.

This book will prove invaluable to any clinician working in the field of Foot and Ankle care including Podiatrists, Podiatric Surgeons, Orthopaedic Surgeons, Rheumatologists, Sports Physicians, Anaesthetists, Pain Specialists, General Practitioners with a special interest, Physiotherapists, and Nurse Specialists. It will act as an important primer for tyro practitioners and an invaluable referral text for even the most experienced clinicians.

Bill Ribbans, PhD, FRCSOrth, FFSEM (UK)
Consultant Trauma and Orthopaedic Surgeon
Visiting Professor, University of Northampton, UK

PREFACE

Some of you will be familiar with Stuart's previous work *Local Anaesthesia for Podiatrists*. Between us we have run injection therapy courses for a number of years and the idea for this book was to update Stuart's work on anaesthesia and incorporate some of our combined knowledge on therapeutic injection therapy.

We have included references and further reading for you to continue your studies but the main thrust of this book is that it is to guide and inform your clinical practice. While there are many concepts freely imparted, the aim of this book is to share some of our practical experience rather than distill the full weight of academic knowledge into a single tome. Some of the concepts remain controversial, for example, the use of corticosteroids in plantar fasciitis. We will discuss theory but in general assume that the decision to inject has already been made. Our hope is to share what, in our experience, has proven to be the best way to do it.

Ian Reilly

CONTENTS

LOCAL ANAESTHETICS 1

HISTORY OF LOCAL ANAESTHESIA

The word anaesthesia is derived from the Greek words "an" – meaning not, without and "aesthetos" – meaning perceptible, able to feel (Askitopoulou et al. 2000). Anaesthesia has traditionally meant the process of blocking the perception of pain and other sensations. Local anaesthesia is a technique used to render part of the body insensitive to pain without affecting consciousness; regional anaesthesia involves a larger part of the body, for example, the foot or arm (Jankovic 2004).

Among the first agents to be used to achieve anaesthesia was ethyl alcohol, which was known to destroy nerve tissue. The first drug successfully used as a local anaesthetic agent was cocaine. Historically it is known that cocaine had been used by natives of Peru for hundreds of years to induce analgesic and hypnotic states. The cocaine was derived from the leaves of the Erythroxylon coca bush, which would be chewed and saliva dropped into the wounds of the patients to reduce pain. Thomas Moreno y Maiz, a Peruvian army surgeon, explored the use of cocaine and published a short paper in 1868 describing experiments using cocaine in which he noted the "numbing"properties of this substance. In 1880 Basil Von Anrep pursued this line of investigation and although producing some successful results with cocaine through self-experimentation, its use was not pursued further by the scientific community for another 5 years (Deschner et al. 2007).

The credit for introducing cocaine as a local anaesthetic has been given to a German ophthalmologist, Carl Koller. Koller, an intern specializing in ophthalmology, working under the guidance of Professor Arit, set about searching for a substance that could be used as a local anaesthetic for the eye. A friend of Koller's, who had developed a morphine addiction following repeated use to control pain, was being treated by Freud (a mutual friend) using cocaine. The use of cocaine to treat such addictions was becoming established at this time. It was this mutual friend, Freud (later to become the famous psychologist), who first provided Koller with some crystals of cocaine. Almost immediately Koller recognized the potential of this substance and tested his ideas first on animals and then on himself. Koller's discovery was reported to the Heidelberg Ophthalmologic Congress on 15 September 1884, whereupon news of this breakthrough was shared with others in the medical community. It is interesting to note that the adverse effects of cocaine were not reported until 1885 by Halsted who produced one of the first papers warning of the addictive properties of cocaine; he himself was an addict. Ironically his addiction was successfully treated using morphine, the very substance that had necessitated treatment by Freud using cocaine (Ball et al. 2003).

The application of local anaesthesia was aided by the development of the hypodermic syringe. The first syringe for human use was patented by Zophar Jayne in 1841. The early successes using cocaine were sadly marred by the now well-recognized complications of this toxic and addictive substance. It is likely that this discovery provided the inspiration to search for alternative drugs that were free of these unwanted effects. This search continued unrewarded until 1904 when Einhorn synthesized procaine, the first ester-type local anaesthetic drug. Not until nearly 40 years later was the first amide-type local anaesthetic synthesized by Löfgren in 1943 (Trent 1946).

The history of regional anaesthesia shows that its development was greatly facilitated by the work of Dr Gaston Labat in the 1920s. Labat developed and refined sophisticated techniques for regional anaesthesia delivery at Bellevue Hospital, New York (Bacon 2002):

> Anatomy is the foundation upon which the entire concept of regional anaesthesia is built. Anyone who wishes to be an expert in the art of regional anaesthesia must be thoroughly grounded in anatomy, for without such knowledge one cannot be successful.

Since that time there has been a continued introduction of newer local anaesthetic drugs in an attempt to produce the "ideal" local anaesthetic combined with technological advancements in equipment and drug delivery. The future for local and regional anaesthesia will see it take an even greater role in the management of our patients.

NERVE PHYSIOLOGY

Higher vertebrates have specialized cells called Schwann cells, which wrap concentric layers of fatty myelin tightly around the nerve axon. The sections of myelin are discontinuous so that periodically along the length of the axon there are regions not covered by myelin sheaths – the nodes of Ranvier (Fig. 1.1). The tight wrapping of myelin prevents any ionic exchange or spread of electric current therefore the action potential can only occur at the nodes.

FIGURE 1.1
Nodes of Ranvier.

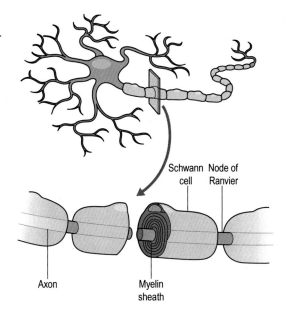

Schwann cell   Node of Ranvier

Axon   Myelin sheath

PLASMA MEMBRANES

Plasma membranes contain specific channels and pumps that control the movement of ions across the membrane (Urban 2002). Ion channels are pore-forming proteins that help to establish and control a voltage gradient across the plasma membrane. The voltage-gated sodium channel is a large complex composed of an alpha subunit and auxiliary beta subunits (Nau & Wang 2004). The channel performs its function as

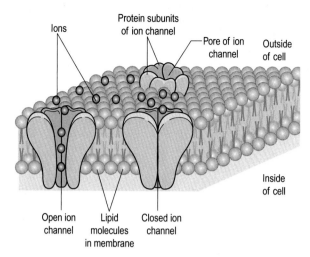

FIGURE 1.2
Ion channels.

a gated conduit for sodium ions (Fig. 1.2) by manifesting three types of gating state (Li et al. 1998):

- closed
- open
- inactivated.

At rest there is a considerable difference between the ion concentration outside and inside the plasma membrane. There is therefore a difference in electrical charges on either side of the membrane. This difference, called a potential difference, is partly the result of an unequal distribution of potassium and sodium ions on either side of the membrane. In resting neurons, the potassium ion concentration inside the cell is about 28–30 times greater than it is outside; the sodium ion concentration is about 14 times greater outside than inside. Other large, non-diffusible negatively charged ions are trapped in the cell. The inside of the membrane is 70 mV less than the outside, that is, the membrane potential is −70 mV.

A stimulus is a change in the environment of sufficient strength to initiate an impulse. If a stimulus of adequate strength is applied to a polarized membrane, the membrane's permeability to sodium ions is greatly increased at the point of stimulation. Sodium channels open and permit the influx of sodium ions by diffusion. Since there are more sodium ions entering than leaving, the electrical potential of the membrane begins to change. The potential inside the membrane changes from −70 mV towards zero. At 0 mV the membrane is said to be depolarized. Some 7000 sodium ions pass through each channel during the brief period (about 1 ms) that it remains open. This initiates the rising phase of the action potential (Yu et al. 2005). Sodium ions continue to rush inside until the membrane potential is reversed (+30 mV). At this point an action potential (nerve impulse) is initiated. Investigators during the last few decades have outlined the voltage-gated sodium channel protein as the prime target for local anaesthetic in mammalian neurons (Scholz 2002).

LOCAL ANAESTHETIC DRUGS

Local anaesthetics are drugs that reversibly block the transmission of nerve impulses. They are used to prevent or reverse acute pain and treat symptoms of chronic pain (Yanagidate 2007). They may be administered by injection, continuous infusion, and some by topical application. Whilst the perfect local anaesthetic does not exist, favourable characteristics include:

- reversibility
- a rapid onset of action
- a predictable duration of action
- good tolerance at high doses with a low risk of systemic toxicity.

Whilst there are many drugs that prevent transmission of an action potential along a nerve, the fundamental property of a local anaesthetic is that of "reversibility."

WHAT ARE LOCAL ANAESTHETICS?

An amine is an organic compound with a functional group that contains nitrogen as the key atom. One, two, or three of the hydrogen atoms can be replaced by other organic units giving rise to primary, secondary, or tertiary amines (Fig. 1.3). Local anaesthetics are classified as amino-amide or amino-esters according to their chemical composition, i.e., type of chemical linkage between the lipophilic and hydrophilic components of the local anaesthetic molecule (Fig. 1.4) (Rosenberg 2000). Ester-type local anaesthetics include amethocaine, benzocaine, cocaine, and procaine and are all hydrolysed by plasma pseudocholinesterases. These agents are derivatives of para-aminobenzoic acid (PABA) and are prone to allergic reaction.

Ester Local Anaesthetics

- Rapidly broken down by pseudocholinesterase
- Derived from PABA thus increased allergy potential

Amino-amides undergo metabolism in the liver and cause fewer allergic reactions than amino-esters (Dullenkopf & Borgeat 2003). This chapter will focus on the amide group of local anaesthetic drugs.

Ester Local Anaesthetics

- Amethocaine
- Benzocaine
- Cocaine
- Procaine

Amide Local Anaesthetics

- Lidocaine
- Prilocaine
- Mepivacaine
- Bupivacaine
- Levobupivacaine
- Ropivacaine

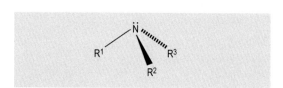

FIGURE 1.3
Tertiary amine.

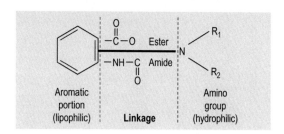

FIGURE 1.4
The basic chemical structure.

STEREOISOMERS

Stereoisomers are isomeric molecules with the same chemical formula but a different atomic arrangement. As a consequence they possess similar chemical and physical properties. Enantiomers are stereoisomers that are chiral (nonsuperimposable mirror images of each other) much as one's left and right hands are the same but opposite (Whiteside & Wildsmith 2001). When compounds exist in different isomeric forms the different molecules can be classified according to their geometry (R for rectus or S for sinister) or the way in which they rotate polarized light: levo for anticlockwise or dextro for clockwise. When the equal amounts of enantiomers are mixed they are termed racemic. Chiral local anaesthetics, such as ropivacaine and levobupivacaine, have the advantage over racemic mixtures in showing reduced systemic toxicity.

PHARMACOKINETICS

Most drugs are either weak acids or weak bases and exist as a mixture of molecules in ionized (charged) and un-ionized forms. The degree of ionization is dependent upon the physiochemical properties of the drug and the environment in which it is located. The pKa (acid dissociation constant) and pH are particularly important. The pKa of a drug molecule is the pH at which the drug is 50% ionized. The relationship between pH, pKa, and percentage ionization is given by the Henderson-Hasselbach equation.

Local anaesthetics are almost insoluble in water. Solubility is greatly increased by preparation of their hydrochloride salts (B·HCl). After injection, the base is liberated by the relatively alkaline pH of tissue fluids:

$$B{\cdot}HCl + HCO_3 \leftrightarrow B + H_2CO_3 + Cl^-$$

In tissue fluid the anaesthetic will be present in both an ionized (BH+) and un-ionized form (B). Movement of anaesthetic molecules occurs by diffusion along a concentration gradient. The un-ionized base (B) (lipid soluble) diffuses through the nerve sheath, perineuronal tissues, and the neuronal membrane to reach the axoplasm.

The pH of the axoplasm is lower than that of the tissue fluid. Once inside the nerve cell (axoplasm), the lower pH results in the molecule being re-ionized, thus inhibiting its passage back out of the cell. This is referred to as "ion-trapping." In the ionized form (BH+), the local anaesthetic blocks the sodium channel and prevents the action potential from being propagated.

How Local Anaesthetics Work

- Local anaesthetic is injected as hydrochloride
- pH increases (tissue pH 7.4), drug dissociates, and free base is released
- Lipid-soluble free base enters the axon
- Inside the axon the pH is lower and thus reionization takes place
- The ionized portion enters the Na$^+$ channel

NERVE SUSCEPTIBILITY TO LOCAL ANAESTHETIC

Small nerve fibres are more sensitive to local anaesthetics than large nerve fibres. Autonomic fibres, small unmyelinated C fibres (mediating pain), and small myelinated A-delta fibres (mediating pain and temperature sensation) are blocked before larger myelinated A-gamma, A-beta, or A-alpha fibres (mediating touch, pressure, muscle, and postural inputs). There is a progressive loss of function as the dose of the local anaesthetic is increased in the order shown in Table 1.1.

Table 1.1 Progressive loss of function as the dose of local anaesthetic increases

TYPE OF NERVE	FUNCTION
C	Pain & temperature
B	Preganglionic autonomic
A-delta	Pain & temperature
A-gamma	Proprioception
A-beta	Touch and pressure
A-alpha	Motor

The variation in nerve susceptibility is a consequence of two factors. Firstly the larger-diameter A fibres are more heavily myelinated than the smaller A-alpha and C fibres. This fatty myelin sheath represents a barrier to diffusion of local anaesthetic molecules. The second factor relates to the greater internodal distance (i.e., the distance between the nodes of Ranvier). Cessation of action potential transmission requires blockade at more than one node as the action potential is able to skip over a single blocked node (Fig. 1.5). Thus, for prevention of action potential propagation a greater length of nerve must be blocked in a large nerve fibre compared with a smaller nerve fibre (Fig. 1.6).

FIGURE 1.5
Number of nodes blocked and propagation.

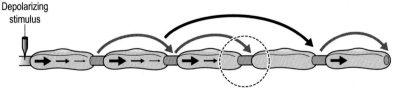

Depolarizing stimulus

Single node blocked and therefore action potential skips and propagation continues

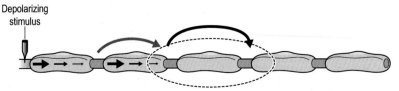

Depolarizing stimulus

Two nodes blocked and therefore action potential cannot skip and conduction ceases

FIGURE 1.6
Small versus large nerve susceptibility to local anaesthetic action.

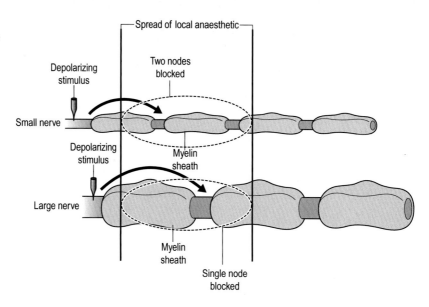

DRUG CHARACTERISTICS

The various local anaesthetic drugs differ in their pharmacological and clinical characteristics. We can summarize the characteristics as:

Local Anaesthetic Characteristics
1 Onset time
2 Duration
3 Distribution
4 Regression
5 Toxicity

Understanding these differences permits the most appropriate drug for a given clinical situation to be selected. It is important to note that in clinical practice many other factors may influence these specific characteristics. For example, bupivacaine is stated as having a longer onset time in comparison to lidocaine. Whilst pharmacologically this is true, when given as a digital block little discernible differences are observed clinically.

ONSET TIME

This is the time taken from the acid dissociation constant. The administration of the anaesthetic to the onset of anaesthesia. The closer the pKa is to local tissue pH (usually 7.4), the more un-ionized the drug is; the higher the pKa, the more ionized it is. Local anaesthetics with a pKa near physiological pH (7.4) will have more molecules in the un-ionized lipid soluble form (e.g., lidocaine) and therefore a more rapid onset of action. At pH 7.4, 35% of lidocaine exists in the un-ionized base form and only 5% of bupivacaine exists in the un-ionized base form.

Low pKa

- More un-ionized molecules
- Better absorption into nerve tissue
- RAPID ONSET BLOCK

High pKa

- More ionized molecules
- Slower entry to the axon
- MORE EFFECTIVE BLOCK

As noted above, the onset of sensory loss will usually precede that of motor loss and thus satisfactory onset times will depend on the desired level of anaesthesia. The degree of myelinization and the distribution of axons within the mixed peripheral nerves will determine the order of anaesthesia for each modality. For example, large heavily myelinated motor nerves will impair penetration of the anaesthetic agent and therefore peripheral axons within each nerve will be reached before those axons located centrally within a mixed peripheral nerve.

Alkalinization

Accelerating onset – elevating the tissue pH by the addition of bicarbonate increases the base:cation ratio thereby increasing absorption of local anaesthetic into nerve

- Onset of PNB may be more rapid in younger patients
- In younger patients the endoneurium is loose and presents less of a barrier to diffusion to local anaesthetic molecules. By virtue of the increased permeability duration may be shorter

DURATION OF ANAESTHESIA (POTENCY)

This is the time between the onset of anaesthesia and the time when the patient begins to appreciate sensory stimuli again. The success of anaesthesia depends on sufficient numbers of local anaesthetic molecules being available to prevent the generation of a nerve impulse. This will depend on the dose of anaesthetic administered and the absorption of these molecules. The duration of anaesthesia depends on a number of drug factors:

- lipid solubility
- molecular size
- protein binding.

Potency is related to lipid solubility. Highly lipid soluble drugs readily cross membranes. The higher the lipid partition coefficient, the more potent and longer the duration of action of the drug. Addition of larger chemical radicals to the amine or aromatic end of a local anaesthetic compound increases its binding to protein. The more highly protein bound the drug, the longer the duration of action. The addition of a vasoconstrictor can prolong the duration of action of a local anaesthetic by decreasing its systemic absorption. Reduced rate of absorption by the addition of a vasoconstrictor is thus associated with a reduction in peak plasma level and enhanced neural blockade.

Potency

Increased lipid solubility – the more lipid-soluble a drug, the more readily it crosses plasma membranes and thus the greater the drug's potency and duration of action

Duration of Action

Increased protein binding – more highly bound, the longer the duration of action. Probably a result of increased binding to neural membranes, which act as a reservoir for molecules

DISTRIBUTION

Distribution of local anaesthetics needs to be considered in the context of local distribution with the tissues at the injection site (i.e., spread) and the systemic distribution within the body. Local anaesthetic solutions are typically introduced via hypodermic syringe and needles or catheter. The spread of local anaesthetic solution within tissues local to the injection site is determined by a number of factors. Initially fluid mechanics are important with the rate/force of injection coupled with volume being most important. The solution will tend to follow the line of least resistance and thus the presence of tissue planes or joint cavities can lead to loss of solution from the desired area.

Local Anaesthetic Spread
- Volume administered
- Vascularity of tissues
- Barriers to diffusion
- Speed of injection
- Forces of injection
- Tissue planes/cavities

An increased volume of anaesthetic drug will increase the spread within tissues though this will not overcome poor injection technique if the needle is placed too far away from the peripheral nerve to be blocked. Rapid injections are associated with increased pain on injection and also risk damage to local tissues. A further problem of rapid and forceful injections is the spread of solution along lines of least resistance into different tissue planes, which can result in loss of solution from the target site. Following this initial deposition, mass movement of anaesthetic molecules is determined by simple diffusion along a concentration gradient. Areas of high vascularity will effectively lose anaesthetic molecules as they are removed to the systemic circulation. This has the effect of reducing local effect and increasing plasma concentration of local anaesthetic.

REGRESSION

This is the time taken from the first appreciation of sensation to complete return of sensory and motor modalities. A long regression period would allow additional time for top-up anaesthesia to be administered from the first signs of sensory return. The regression time of an anaesthetic is determined by its receptor affinity and its effects on tissue perfusion. Drugs with greater vasodilatory properties will therefore have shorter regression times.

TOXICITY

This literally means "poisonous" and refers to the presence of "unwanted" effects as a result of the administration of a given dose of drug. Side effects are the effects that are clinically undesirable. Local anaesthetics are amphipathic compounds meaning that they possess both hydrophilic and hydrophobic properties. As such they are able to cross plasma and intracellular membranes interacting with a wide range of cellular processes. Therefore toxic effects are seen in a wide variety of tissues including heart, brain, and skeletal muscle. There are substantial differences in the relative toxicities of the various local anaesthetic drugs. Bupivacaine is the most cardiotoxic of all of the amide local anaesthetics and has been associated with the most fatalities in clinical practice.

Whilst many of the toxic effects associated with local anaesthetics are believed to be mediated by their interactions with voltage-gated sodium channels, at high doses local anaesthetics can disrupt every metabotropic and ionotropic neurotransmitter receptor. Bupivacaine especially interferes with oxidative phosphorylation depleting cells of essential energy (via reduced ATP synthesis). These observations coincide with the clinical features of acute local anaesthetic toxicity in which those tissues with greatest aerobic demand and least intolerance for hypoxia are affected first. Clinically toxicity is usually heralded by initial central nervous system (CNS) features later to be followed by cardiac arrhythmias and myocardial depression.

Plasma concentration of local anaesthetics following administration depends on many factors including total dose, protein binding, route of administration, and rate of absorption. Peak plasma levels are typically reached approximately 30 minutes after administration. Toxicity from administration of local anaesthetics usually arises from either intravascular injection or exceeding the recommended safe dose.

LIDOCAINE HYDROCHLORIDE

Please refer to Table 1.2 for the properties of lidocaine hydrochloride.

Table 1.2 Lidocaine hydrochloride

Chemistry	$C_{14}H_{12}N_2O \cdot HCl$ 2-(diethylamino)-N-(2,6-dimethylphenyl)acetamide
Brand name	Xylocaine
General	Lidocaine hydrochloride was synthesized by Löfgren and Lundquist in 1943, and was clinically introduced in 1948. It remains one of the most widely used local anaesthetics. It can be administered parenterally for a peripheral nerve block (PNB), intravenously, or applied topically at strengths of 2–4%. The addition of epinephrine 1:200000 to 1:100000 slows the vascular absorption of lidocaine and prolongs its effects

Table 1.2 Lidocaine hydrochloride—cont'd

Available concentrations	0.5%
	1% with/without epinephrine 1/200 000
	2% with/without epinephrine 1/200 000
	4% (topical)
	5% (medicated plaster)
Dose mg/kg	3 (without epinephrine)
	7 (with epinephrine)
Additional dose guidelines	600 mg by topical application in 24 h
	200 mg for PNB
	500 mg for PNB (with epinephrine)
	Elderly: doses may need to be reduced depending on age and physical state
Onset time	Fast (2–5 min)
Duration of anaesthesia	Short (45–60 min)
Peak plasma levels	15–30 min
Relative toxicity	Low: 1
	(toxicity values for the other drugs will be compared to lidocaine)
Mean half life	1.5 hr
Protein binding	65–75%
Volume of distribution	90 L
Metabolism	Lidocaine is metabolized by the liver with only a small amount (3%) found unchanged in urine. The three main mechanisms of metabolism are shown below:
	N-de-ethylation > monoethylglycinexylidide (MEGX) > glycinexylidide
	Hydrolysis of glycinexylidide
	5-hydroxylation of lidocaine's benzene ring
	Lidocaine possesses convulsant activity. Hepatic disease or reduced hepatic blood flow (as in congestive cardiac failure) will lower metabolic capacity
Potency	Medium
Excretion	Renal
Relative lipid solubility	150
pKa	7.86
Drug interactions	Cimetidine – inhibits hepatic metabolism
	Propranolol – reduces systemic clearance by up to 40% by reducing hepatic metabolism
Additional information	Lidocaine is contraindicated in patients with known hypersensitivity to local anaesthetics of the amide type and in patients with porphyria. Reactions due to overdose with lidocaine (high plasma levels) are systemic and involve the central nervous and cardiovascular systems. Effects include medullary depression, tonic and clonic convulsions, and cardiovascular collapse
	Solutions in multidose vials may contain hydrobenzoate derivatives and have been associated with allergic reactions in some patients. As with all of the amide local anaesthetics protein binding is reduced in the neonate (50% versus 64% in the adult), which necessitates reduced doses if adverse reactions are to be avoided

PRILOCAINE HYDROCHLORIDE

Please refer to Table 1.3 for the properties of prilocaine hydrochloride.

Table 1.3 Prilocaine hydrochloride

Chemistry	$C_{13}H_{20}N_2O \cdot HCl$ N-(2-methylphenyl)-2-propylamino-propanamide
Brand name	Citanest
Available concentrations	1–4% Lower concentrations are only suitable for local infiltration techniques. For PNBs either 2% or 4% solutions should be utilized
Dose mg/kg	6
Additional dose guidelines	The maximum dose for healthy adults should not exceed 400 mg
Onset time	Medium (10 min)
Duration of anaesthesia	Medium (120–180 min)
Peak plasma levels	10–20 min
Relative toxicity	Low:1
Mean half life	1–2 h
Protein binding	40–55%
Volume of distribution	156 L
Metabolism	Extra hepatic sites (lung & kidney) play a significant role in the metabolism of prilocaine although the liver remains the major site. Prilocaine has the highest volume of distribution of all the local anaesthetics and because of these two features the risk of toxicity is lowest with this amide anaesthetic One of the metabolites of prilocaine, hydroxytoluidine, is able to reduce haemoglobin to form methaemoglobin, which is unable to transport oxygen. Although methaemoglobinaemia is only associated with large doses of prilocaine (>600 mg) this drug is specifically contraindicated in patients with severe anaemia or methaemoglobinaemia because of the risk of exacerbating either of these clinical conditions
Potency	Medium
Excretion	Renal
Relative lipid solubility	50

Table 1.3 Prilocaine hydrochloride—cont'd

pKa	7.9
Drug interactions	Ester local anaesthetics: prilocaine is a potent inhibitor of cholinesterase (metabolism of ester-type anaesthetics)
Additional information	Prilocaine hydrochloride should be avoided in pregnancy as foetal haemoglobin is more sensitive to the development of methaemoglobinaemia and, as with other amide local anaesthetics, is able to cross from the maternal to the foetal circulation. Concurrent administration of ester-type local anaesthetics should be avoided as prilocaine is a potent inhibitor of cholinesterase, which is responsible for the metabolism of ester anaesthetics. Concurrent administration increases the risk of toxicity from the ester anaesthetic
	There were a limited number of reports of local skin necrosis at the injection sites following digital blocks using 4% prilocaine hydrochloride (Citanest) in the late 1990s. There appears to be little evidence that this was a complication of the drug per se. It is possible that these few reports relate to instances where excessive volumes had been administered causing local pressure necrosis of tissues at the injection site

MEPIVACAINE HYDROCHLORIDE

Please refer to Table 1.4 for the properties of mepivacaine hydrochloride.

Table 1.4 Mepivacaine hydrochloride

Chemistry	$C_{15}H_{22}N_2O\cdot HCl$ N-(2,6-dimethylphenyl)-1-methyl-piperidine-2-carboxamide
Brand name	Scandonest
General	Mepivacaine was the second amide local anaesthetic to be clinically introduced. Mepivacaine, together with bupivacaine and ropivacaine, was synthesized by Ekenstam in the 1950s
Available concentrations	1%–3% Concentrations of less than 3% are of little value in PNBs
Dose mg/kg	6
Additional dose guidelines	The maximum dose for healthy adults should not exceed 400 mg
Onset time	Medium (10 min)
Duration of anaesthesia	Medium (120–180 min)
Peak plasma levels	10–20 min

Continued

Table 1.4 Mepivacaine hydrochloride—cont'd

Relative toxicity	Low: 1.4
Mean half life	1–2 h
Protein binding	8%
Volume of distribution	156 L
Metabolism	Liver
Potency	Medium
Excretion	Renal
Relative lipid solubility	50
pKa	7.9
Additional information	Mepivacaine has been shown to be less toxic (systemic and neural tissue) than lidocaine in adults and provides a somewhat longer duration of action than lidocaine because of a less pronounced vasodilatory effect

BUPIVACAINE HYDROCHLORIDE

Please refer to Table 1.5 for the properties of bupivacaine hydrochloride.

Table 1.5 Bupivacaine hydrochloride

Chemistry	$C_{18}H_{28}N_2O \cdot HCl$ 1-butyl-*N*-(2,6dimethylphenyl)piperidine-2-carboxamide
Brand name	Marcain
General	The most potent of the amide local anaesthetics. Used in concentrations between 0.25% and 0.5% for local infiltrations and PNBs, respectively. It has a much longer duration of action than many of the other local anaesthetics (Green et al. 1979)
Available concentrations	0.25% 0.5%
Dose mg/kg	2
Additional dose guidelines	The recommended maximum single dose is 150 mg. Where sustained motor and sensory block are required for a prolonged procedure, additional doses may be required. The maximum recommended dose during a 24-h period is 400 mg. For post-operative pain management, the dose should not exceed 18.75 mg/h

Table 1.5 Bupivacaine hydrochloride—cont'd

Onset time	15–30 min Local factors are also important and for digital anaesthesia onset is rapid
Duration of anaesthesia	8–16 h
Peak plasma levels	10–20 min
Relative toxicity	High: 4. It is the most cardiotoxic of all the local anaesthetics and is contraindicated for use in intravenous anaesthesia due to the risk of cardiotoxicity. Toxicity as a result of bupivacaine administration is significantly more resistant to management than with other local anaesthetic agents. This may be a result of both the receptor affinity (slow in slow out) and the effect on other cellular processes such as oxidative phosphorylation leading to ATP depletion
Mean half life	2.7 h
Protein binding	95%
Volume of distribution	73 L
Metabolism	Liver
Potency	High
Excretion	Renal
Relative lipid solubility	1000
pKa	7.6
Drug interactions	Ester local anaesthetics: bupivacaine is a potent inhibitor of cholinesterase (metabolism of ester-type anaesthetics)
Additional information	Bupivacaine is contraindicated in intravenous regional anaesthesia. Bupivacaine has been reported to cause an unpleasant stinging sensation when administered for peripheral nerve blocks. The duration of anaesthesia is not increased significantly by the addition of a vasoconstrictor

LEVOBUPIVACAINE

Historically there have been several cases of severe cardiotoxicity (including death) reported in association with the administration of bupivacaine. Racemic bupivacaine exists as levobupivacaine (the S-enantiomer) and dextrobupivacaine (the R-enantiomer). Although the enantiomers of bupivacaine possess identical physiochemical properties, the pharmacological and toxicity effects on the body are different because of key stereoselective differences in binding of the drug to its receptor site. Dextrobupivacaine exhibits a "fast in; slow out" blockade of cardiac sodium channels whereas levobupivacaine demonstrates a "fast in; fast out" block (Valenzuela et al. 1995). Compared to the levo-enantiomer, dextrobupivacaine binds three times more firmly to the sodium channels and is released over four times more slowly, which accounts for the increased toxicity. The two drugs have a similar partial coefficient but levobupivacaine has a longer duration of action than bupivacaine and produces less vasodilatation (Foster & Markham 2000).

Observations that the *R*-isomer component of bupivacaine had a higher potential for toxicity led researchers to consider whether a drug containing only the levorotatory isomer might be associated with a reduced risk for cardiac toxicity and neurotoxicity. This assumption proved to be correct and the preparation of levobupivacaine, which contains only the levorotatory isomer, retains the anaesthetic characteristics of bupivacaine with the advantage of reduced toxicity. The *S*-enantiomer (levobupivacaine) has therefore been developed for clinical use. Foster and Markham reviewed preclinical and toxicity data, reporting an advantage of levobupivacaine over bupivacaine. There would appear to be little justifiable reason to continue using bupivacaine when levobupivacaine and ropivacaine offer the same anaesthetic characteristics with reduced toxicity (Uddin 2008).

Please refer to Table 1.6 for the properties of levobupivacaine hydrochloride.

Table 1.6 Levobupivacaine hydrochloride

Chemistry	$C_{18}H_{28}N_2O \cdot HCl$ (S)1-butyl-*N*-(2,6dimethylphenyl)piperidine-2-carboxamide
Brand name	Chirocaine
Available concentrations	2.5, 5.0,7.5 mg/mL in 10-mL ampoules
Dose mg/kg	2
Additional dose guidelines	The recommended maximum single dose is 150 mg. Where sustained motor and sensory block are required for a prolonged procedure, additional doses may be required. The maximum recommended dose during a 24-h period is 400 mg. For post-operative pain management, the dose should not exceed 18.75 mg/h Field block 1–60 mL (max 150 mg) of 2.5 mg/mL solution PNB 1–40 mL of 2.5 mg/mL or 5 mg/mL solution
Onset time	Slow
Duration of anaesthesia	Long
Peak plasma levels	20 min
Relative toxicity	Medium: 3
Mean half life	80 ± 22 h

Table 1.6 Levobupivacaine hydrochloride—cont'd

Protein binding	95%
Volume of distribution	67 L
Metabolism	Extensively metabolized with no unchanged drug detected in the urine or faeces
Potency	High
Excretion	71% urine 24% faeces
Relative lipid solubility	1000
pKa	8.1

ROPIVACAINE HYDROCHLORIDE

Ropivacaine is the most recently introduced amide local anaesthetic drug and was developed by AstraZeneca to address the issues of toxicity associated with bupivacaine. Ropivacaine is manufactured as a pure S-enantiomer in order to take advantage of the decreased cardiotoxicity of the S-configuration, the S-enantiomer being less firmly held at the sodium channels than the R-enantiomer. As a consequence ropivacaine is significantly less cardiotoxic than bupivacaine. In fact in a study designed to assess acute central nervous and cardiovascular toxicity in humans, ropivacaine caused less CNS symptoms and was at least 25% less toxic than bupivacaine in regard to the dose tolerated (Scott et al. 1989). Other researchers have confirmed similar reductions in toxicity in a range of animal studies (Nancarrow et al. 1989; Feldman et al. 1991). These differences in toxicity between ropivacaine and bupivacaine roughly parallel the reported anaesthetic potency ratio of these two drugs.

Like the other amide local anaesthetics ropivacaine is metabolized by the liver and excreted via the kidneys. Clearance of the intact drug accounts for a minor proportion of total clearance. Peak plasma levels of ropivacaine following epidural or peripheral nerve block (PNB) may rise twice as high as levels of bupivacaine, likely due to ropivacaine's decreased lipid solubility and volume of distribution (Datta et al. 1995).

Clinical trials comparing bupivacaine and ropivacaine in epidural and axillary block demonstrate similar potency with respect to the intensity of sensory anaesthesia (Brockway et al. 1991; Hickey et al. 1991, 1992). Motor block with ropivacaine, however, may be delayed in onset, less intense, and shorter in duration compared with bupivacaine – this is because it is less lipophilic (Brockway et al. 1991; de Jong 1995; Beaulieu et al. 2006). Maintenance of sensory blockade without prolonged motor loss has a number of key benefits in ambulatory surgery where loss of motor power might, for example, mandate longer periods of hospitalization.

The addition of a vasoconstrictor to ropivacaine does not appear to significantly increase the mean duration of action in either epidural or PNBs (Hickey & Candido 1990). Ropivacaine is itself vasoconstrictive and the addition of epinephrine does not increase the level of vasoconstriction.

Please refer to Table 1.7 for the properties of ropivacaine hydrochloride.

Table 1.7 Ropivacaine hydrochloride

Chemistry	$C_{17}H_{26}N_2O \cdot HCl$ S)-N-(2,6-dimethylphenyl)-1-propylpiperidine-2-carboxamide
Brand name	Naropin
Available concentrations	0.2%, 0.5%, 0.75%, 1%
Dose mg/kg	4.5 Continuous peripheral nerve block 700 mg/24 h by slow infusion

Additional dose guidelines	Field block
	  • 30 mL of 7.5mg/mL solution
	  • 100 mL of 2 mg/mL solution
	PNB
	  • 5–10 mL/h of 2 mg/mL by infusion or intermittent injection

Onset time	Slow (15–30 min)
Duration of anaesthesia	Long
Peak plasma levels	10–20 min
Relative toxicity	Medium: 3. 25% less than bupivacaine
Mean half life	111 min
Protein binding	94%
Volume of distribution	41 L
Metabolism	Liver
Potency	High
Excretion	Renal
Relative lipid solubility	400
pKa	8.1
Drug interactions	There is a potential risk for metabolic interaction when ropivacaine is used in combination with CYP1A-inhibitors such as verapamil, which may result in increased plasma levels
Additional information	Ropivacaine is moderately vasoconstrictive Duration of action unaffected by addition of vasoconstrictor

EMLA CREAM

EMLA refers to the "eutectic mixture of local anaesthetic" and contains two active ingredients, lidocaine and prilocaine. Each gram of cream contains 25 mg of lidocaine and 25 mg of prilocaine. It is a topical local anaesthetic agent that has a limited range of clinical applications in the lower limb. The serendipitous discovery was that this compound has a melting point of 16 °C and is a liquid at room temperature with the individual components as crystalline solids, with a high base content. It takes 50 minutes to achieve its maximum effect.

Please refer to Table 1.8 for the properties of EMLA.

Table 1.8 EMLA

Brand name	EMLA
Available concentrations	50% lidocaine hydrochloride and 50% prilocaine hydrochloride. Each gram contains 25 mg lidocaine and 25 mg of prilocaine in a eutectic mixture as an oil–water emulsion
Dose	For skin apply a thick layer of cream under an occlusive dressing. 2 g EMLA for a minimum of 60 min
Use	Minor dermatological procedures Venous and arterial cannulation Lumbar puncture Drug reservoir injections EMG needle insertion Superficial skin suturing Otitis externa Postherpetic neuralgia
Onset time	Apply 60 min prior to procedure to a maximum of 5 h
Duration of anaesthesia	2–3 h
Peak plasma levels	3–6 h
Use in pregnancy	Both drugs cross the placental barrier. However, both drugs have been in widespread clinical use for many years and a large number of women have been exposed with no known specific effects on the foetus
Use in breast-feeding	See pregnancy
Metabolism	Liver
Interactions	There is a theoretical potential of methaemoglobinaemia due to prilocaine and its metabolite o-toluidine
Additional information	Swallowing the ointment – anaesthesia of upper airway with loss of protective reflexes Local reactions Vasoconstriction – pallor Oedema Itching Rash Methaemoglobinaemia Toxicity

AMETOP

Ametop (tetracaine 4%) is another widely used topical local anaesthetic agent with similar indications to EMLA cream but which has an "ester" rather than "amide" active ingredient.

Please refer to Table 1.9 for the properties of Ametop.

Table 1.9 Ametop

Brand name	Ametop
Available concentrations	4% tetracaine w/v
Dose mg/kg	Adults and children over 5 y may receive a maximum of 5 tubes (5 g) at different sites at any one time
Use	Percutaneous local anaesthetic to produce anaesthesia of the skin prior to venepuncture or venous cannulation. Apply the contents of the tube to the centre of the area to be anaesthetized and cover with an occlusive dressing. The contents expellable from 1 tube (approximately 1 g) are sufficient to cover and anaesthetize an area of up to 30 cm^2 (6 x 5 cm). Smaller areas of anaesthetized skin may be adequate in infants and small children
Onset time	Apply 30–45 min prior to procedure
Duration of anaesthesia	4–6 h
Peak plasma levels	3–6 h
Use in pregnancy	No specific information as to the safety of tetracaine in pregnancy and breast-feeding; however the drug has been in use for many years without known adverse events. The rapid hydrolysis by plasma cholinesterase suggests when used correctly it should present no risk to the foetus
Use in breast-feeding	It is not known whether tetracaine or its metabolites are secreted in breast milk and therefore the drug is not recommended in breast-feeding mothers
Metabolism	Metabolized in tissues by plasma cholinesterase
Excretion	n/a
Interactions	None known
Additional information	Each tube is intended for use on a single occasion only Topical, white, opalescent gel, each gram containing 40 mg of tetracaine base Not recommended for infants under 1 month Do not apply to broken skin or mucous membranes Other excipients: • Sodium hydroxide • Sodium methyl-*p*-hydroxybenzoate • Sodium propyl-*p*-hydroxybenzoate • Monobasic potassium phosphate • Xanthan gum • Sodium chloride • Purified water

REFERENCES

Askitopoulou, H., Ramoutsaki, I.A., Konsolaki, E., 2000. Analgesia and anesthesia: etymology and literary history of related Greek words. Anesth. Analg. 91, 486–491.

Bacon, D.R., Labat, G., Lundy, J., Rovenstine, E., the Mayo Clinic, 2002. The spread of regional anesthesia in America between the World Wars. J. Clin. Anaesthesiol. 14, 315–320.

Ball, C., Westhorpe, R., 2003. Local anaesthesia – Freud, Koller and cocaine. Anaesth. Intensive Care 31 (3), 249.

Beaulieu, P., Babin, D., Hemmerling, T., 2006. The pharmacodynamics of ropivacaine and bupivacaine in combined sciatic and femoral nerve blocks for total knee arthroplasty. Anesth. Analg. 103, 768–774.

Brockway, M.S., Bannister, J., McClure, J.H., et al., 1991. Comparison of extradural ropivacaine and bupivacaine. Br. J. Anaesth. 66, 31–37.

Datta, S., Camann, W., Bader, A., et al., 1995. Clinical effects and maternal and foetal plasma concentrations of epidural ropivacaine versus bupivacaine for cesarean section. Anesthesiology 82, 1346–1352.

de Jong, R.H., 1995. Garston Labat Lecture: ropivacaine: white knight or dark horse? Region Anaesth. 20, 474–481.

Deschner, B., Robards, C., Somasundaram, L., Harrop-Griffiths, W., 2007. The history of local anaesthesia. In: Hadžić, A. (Ed.), The Textbook of Regional Anaesthesia and Acute Pain Management. McGraw Medical, New York, pp. 3–18.

Dullenkopf, A., Borgeat, A., 2003. Local anaesthetics: differences and similarities in the -cains. Anaesthetist 52, 329–340.

Feldman, H.S., Arthur, G.R., Pitkanen, M., et al., 1991. Treatment of acute systemic toxicity after the rapid intravenous injection of ropivacaine and bupivacaine in the conscious dog. Anesth. Analg. 73, 373–384.

Foster, R.H., Markham, A., 2000. Levobupivacaine: a review of its pharmacology and use as a local anaesthetic. Drugs 59, 551–579.

Hickey, R., Candido, K.D., Ramamurthy, S., et al., 1990. Brachial plexus block with a new local anaesthetic: 0.5 per cent ropivacaine. Can. J. Anaesth. 37, 732–738.

Hickey, R., Hoffman, J., Ramamurthy, S., Rossignoli, L., 1991. A comparison of ropivacaine 0.5% and bupivacaine 0.5% for brachial plexus block. Anesthesiology 74, 639–642.

Hickey, R., Rowley, C.L., Candido, K.D., et al., 1992. A comparative study of 0.25% ropivacaine and 0.25% bupivacaine for brachial plexus block. Anesth. Analg. 75, 602–606.

Jankovic, D., 2004. Regional Nerve Blocks and Infiltration Therapy. A Textbook and Colour Atlas, third ed. Blackwell Publishing Ltd, Berlin, pp. 10–14.

Li, H.L., Galue, A., Meadows, L., Ragsdale, D.S., 1998. A molecular basis for the different local anesthetic affinities of resting versus open and inactivated states of the sodium channel. Mol. Pharmacol. 55, 134–141.

Nancarrow, C., Rutten, A.J., Runciman, W.B., et al., 1989. Myocardial and cerebral drug concentrations and the mechanisms of death after fatal intravenous doses of lidocaine, bupivacaine, and ropivacaine in sheep. Anesth. Analg. 69, 276–283.

Nau, C., Wang, G.K., 2004. Interactions of local anesthetics with voltage-gated Na^+ channels. J. Membr. Biol. 201, 1–8.

Rosenberg, P., 2000. Local and Regional Anaesthesia. BMJ Books Limited, Cornwall.

Scholz, A., 2002. Mechanisms of (local) anaesthetics on voltage-gated sodium and other ion channels. Br. J. Anaesth. 89, 52–61.

Scott, D.B., Lee, A., Fagan, D., et al., 1989. Acute toxicity of ropivacaine compared with that of bupivacaine. Anesth. Analg. 69, 563–569.

Trent, J., 1946. Surgical anesthesia, 1846-1946. J. Hist. Med. Allied Sci. 1, 505–514.

Uddin, A., Reilly, I., 2008. Ropivacaine and levobupivacaine: new drugs for podiatric medicine and surgery. Podiatry Now 11, 22–28.

Urban, B.W., 2002. Current assessment of targets and theories of anaesthesia. Br. J. Anaesth. 89, 167–183.

Valenzuela, C., Delpon, E., Tamkun, M.M., et al., 1995. Stereoselective block of a human cardiac potassium channel (Kv1.5) by bupivacaine enantiomers. Biophys. J. 69, 418–427.

Whiteside, J.B., Wildsmith, J.A.W., 2001. Developments in local anaesthetic drugs. Br. J. Anaesth. 87, 27–35.

Yanagidate, F., Strichartz, G.R., 2007. Local anesthetics. Handb. Exp. Pharmacol. 177, 95–127.

Yu, F.H., Yarovoy, V.Y., Gutman, G.A., Catterall, W.A., 2005. Overview of molecular relationship in the voltage-gated ion channel superfamily. Pharmacol. Rev. 57, 387–395.

BIBLIOGRAPHY AND FURTHER READING

Butterworth, J.F. 4th, Strichartz, G.R., 1990. Molecular mechanisms of local anesthesia: a review. Anesthesiology 72, 711–734.

Haas, D.A., Carmichael, F.J.L., 2007. Local Anaesthetics in Principles of Medical Pharmacology, seventh ed. Elsevier, Canada, pp. 266–274.

Knudsen, K., Suurkula, M.B., Blomberg, S., et al., 1997. Central nervous and cardiovascular effects of i.v infusions of ropivacaine, bupivacaine and placebo in volunteers. Br J Anaesth 78, 507–514.

Lipkind, G.M., Fozzard, H.A., 2005. Molecular modelling of local anesthetic drug binding by voltage-gated sodium channels. Mol. Pharmacol. 68, 1611–1622.

Marban, E., Yamagishi, T., Tomaselli, F., 1998. Structure and function of voltage-gated sodium channels. J. Physiol. 508, 647–657.

McClure, J.H., 1996. Ropivacaine. Br. J. Anaesth. 76, 300–307.

Morrison, L.M.M., Emanuelsson, B.M., McClure, J.H., et al., 1994. Efficacy and kinetics of extradural ropivacaine: comparison with bupivacaine. Br. J. Anaesth. 72, 164–169.

Rang, H.P., Dale, M.M., Ritter, J.M., Flower, R.J., 2007. Pharmacology. Local Anaesthetics and other Drugs Affecting Sodium Channels. Churchill Livingstone, China.

Sheets, M.F., Hanck, D.A., 2003. Molecular action of lidocaine on the voltage sensors of sodium channels. J. Gen. Physiol. 121, 163–175.

Tuttle, A.A., Katz, J.A., Bridenbaugh, P.O., et al., 1995. A double-blind comparison of the abdominal wall relaxation produced by epidural 0.75% ropivacaine and 0.75% bupivacaine in gynecologic surgery. Reg. Anesth. 20, 515–520.

Vegh, V., Cizmarik, J., Hahnenkamp, K., 2006. Is there a place for local anesthetics structurally different from classical amid or ester local anaesthetics? Curr. Opin. Anaesthesiol. 19, 509–515.

APPLICATIONS OF LOCAL ANAESTHETICS 2

SELECTING A LOCAL ANAESTHETIC

Local anaesthetics should be selected based upon their particular characteristics in terms of onset time, duration of action, potency, toxicity, motor power loss, and effect on the local vascularity. In practical terms onset times differ very little and often it is the nature of the block that will influence onset more than the drug used. A good example is when undertaking a digital block with bupivacaine; onset of anaesthesia is rapid. In contrast a popliteal PNB with lidocaine will not take effect in the stated 5 minutes.

> **Considerations when Selecting a Local Anaesthetic**
> - Onset time
> - Duration of action
> - Vasoconstriction
> - Motor block
> - Concentration
> - Toxicity
> - Specific contraindications

For surgical anaesthesia of the lower limb there would seem little value in selecting a short-acting local anaesthetic agent. Short-acting drugs are more applicable to other clinical applications such as diagnostic nerve blocks or joint injections where rapid recovery may be desirable so that the impact of the block can be investigated without undue delay. Some drugs such as bupivacaine and levobupivacaine are specifically contraindicated for intravenous regional anaesthesia, and drugs with least relative toxicity are preferred, i.e., prilocaine.

Where motor blockade is specifically sought a lipophilic agent at a higher concentration is preferred. This is because A-alpha motor fibres are heavily myelinated and the more lipophilic the drug the more readily it is able to diffuse into the nerve. The increased diameter of these A-alpha fibres and greater internodal distances (distance between the nodes of Ranvier) necessitate both increased spread of solution and a greater number of available anaesthetic molecules to facilitate motor block.

CLINICAL APPLICATIONS OF LOCAL ANAESTHETICS

Over the last two decades there has been a rapid increase in the application of local anaesthetics in clinical practice. There are many factors that have contributed to this increase in use. Recognition of the value of neuroaxial blockade in enhancing haemodynamic stability of patients during surgery has favoured an increase in the use of PNBs during surgery, even when general anaesthesia is applied. Development of newer and safer local anaesthetic agents such as ropivacaine and levobupivacaine has provided the opportunity for prolonged post-operative analgesia with reduced risks of toxicity. Technological advances in equipment such as nerve stimulators and more recently high-definition ultrasound have further paved the way for improvements in PNB techniques and thus block reliability. In the context of global healthcare it should also be noticed that there has been a notable shift in the types of surgeries undertaken with local anaesthesia in place of more traditional methods. This appears to have found favour with both patients and government alike at a time of rising cost burden of healthcare provision across the world. Many subspeciality services have started to perform PNBs themselves, such as in ophthalmology, podiatry, and dentistry. This can represent not only direct manpower savings but has seen a crossing of professional boundaries.

Factors Contributing to Rising Applications of Local Anaesthesia
- Haemodynamic stability with neuroaxial blocks
- Safer drugs, e.g., levobupivacaine/ropivacaine
- Post-operative analgesia
- Pre-emptive analgesia
- Enhanced techniques/training
- Policy – day case surgery

Local anaesthetics have many applications in medicine and surgery. In the context of this book we will focus on the use of local anaesthetics in the management of lower limb pathology, which include the following:

Applications of Local Anaesthetics
- Surgery
- Pain control
- Diagnostic local anaesthetic blocks
- Joint MUA
- Pre-emptive analgesia

SURGICAL ANAESTHESIA

In 1846 William T. G. Morton undertook the first successful demonstration of ether anaesthesia in the Massachusetts General Hospital, Boston, USA. This was rapidly embraced by the medical communities of the day and general anaesthesia became the norm for surgical procedures for many years. Only recently has interest in alternative techniques such as peripheral nerve blocks developed. To this day despite an excellent safety record, local anaesthesia has yet to gain universal acceptance by surgeons performing lower limb surgery. Improved understanding, better local anaesthetic drugs, and refined techniques in combination with economic pressures have gone some way to driving the increase in the utilization of local anaesthesia in 21st century medicine and surgery.

Where patient anxiety is a barrier to surgery under local anaesthetic alone, combination with sedatives/anxiolytics provides a useful "middle ground" in the form of conscious sedation and local anaesthetic. This technique has greatly extended the application of local anaesthetic techniques, particularly in the field of ambulatory lower limb surgery. In deciding whether PNB is an appropriate technique the following considerations are useful:

Suitability for Surgery with Local Anaesthetics
- Contraindications to local anaesthetic drugs
- Patient psychological suitability
- Age of the patient
- Ability to achieve anaesthesia of limb
- Tourniquet requirements

Allergy to amide local anaesthetic drugs though rare would constitute an obvious barrier to their safe use. Some patients are enthusiastic about the opportunity to avoid a general anaesthetic for their proposed intervention, while others express concern regarding being conscious during the procedure. A thorough and honest discussion regarding what is involved with a particular procedure, including the PNB itself, is essential. Young children should be counselled very carefully and in most instances a general anaesthetic remains the gold standard, minimizing distress for both parent and child. In lower extremity surgery tourniquet application affords improved visualization and thus an easier operating environment. Surgeries requiring thigh tourniquet are not feasible using PNB technique and spinal or general anaesthesia is necessary in such cases.

Local Anaesthetic Blocks for Common Surgical Procedures

Local infiltration
- Isolated skin lesions
- Small subcutaneous lesions

Digital
- Nail surgery
- Removal of digital exostoses

Isolated tibial
- Surgery to plantar of the foot not involving osseous structure

Ankle
- Any forefoot and midfoot surgery

Popliteal + saphenous
- Any surgical procedure involving structures below the level of the knee

---

PAIN CONTROL

CURRENT STATUS OF POST-OPERATIVE PAIN MANAGEMENT

Undertreatment of post-operative pain remains very common despite improved understanding of effective strategies and newer medicines and technologies. Carr and co-workers demonstrated post-operative pain management to be inadequately managed in over 50% of surgical procedures (Carr & Goudas 1999). In a review of pain management Scott and colleagues found that over 50% of patients at discharge felt their instructions about post-operative pain management were either "unclear" or "nonexistent". Despite this, 80% of the same patient group were satisfied with their pain management. It might be that whilst all healthcare workers agree that, in theory, we should adopt integrated strategies to ensure minimal post-operative pain, clinicians and patients have an almost inherent acceptance that surgery will be followed by the experience of post-operative pain. The previously accepted view that "breakthrough" pain followed most if not all surgical procedures is outdated and the strategy of waiting for and then managing this is ineffective (Kuhn 1990). Post-operative pain management is further complicated by the variability of pain perception to each individual making it necessary to tailor pain management plans to patients and not procedures. In today's healthcare economy such integrated approaches can be difficult to justify on economic grounds alone.

Despite the individuality of pain perception it may however be possible to stratify certain groups so as to introduce appropriate management strategies. There is some evidence to suggest that patients with known anxiety may report higher levels of post-operative pain. Procedure length has been associated with increased post-operative pain as have orthopaedic procedures (bone surgery) and painful prior experiences.

RISK FACTORS FOR INCREASED PAIN

- Previous painful experiences
- Patient anxiety
- Increased operating time
- Orthopaedic surgery

IMPACT OF INADEQUATE PAIN MANAGEMENT

Inadequate pain management has two key consequences: (1) the impact of immediate unpleasantness of the experience; and (2) the potential of modulation of response to future noxious stimuli. At its worst this amplification can lead to otherwise non-noxious stimuli being perceived as pain (hyperalgesia) with the potential for the development of chronic pain syndromes. More generally we know that inadequate pain management has both immediate and longer lasting implications. Control of post-operative pain is a major determinant of wound oxygen tensions, which have a direct impact on the risk of surgical wound infection (Akca et al. 1999). Prior painful experiences are a predictor of increased analgesic use in future surgery (Bachiocco et al. 1993).

PAIN PERCEPTION

Post-operative pain is generated by two distinct components. First the initial surgical insult leads to immediate stimulation of nociceptors, which is followed by generation of inflammatory stimuli via the release of various chemical mediators in response to tissue injury. Though a detailed discussion of the complex mechanisms underpinning pain perception and modulation is beyond the remit of this short text, a brief review is useful for putting into context the role of local anaesthetics in the management of post-operative pain.

Perception of pain involves both the peripheral and central nervous systems. Application of a noxious stimulus leads to activation of peripheral nociceptors, which in turn generates an action potential within the afferent pain fibres (primarily small myelinated A and unmyelinated C fibres). This "pain signal" is conducted from the periphery along these afferent nerve fibres to the spinal cord. Within the spinal cord, pain signals are then conducted along the spinothalamic tract to the thalamus and sensory cortex of the brain. Modulation of the pain signal can occur by a variety of mechanisms including input from both other sensory pathways and descending spinal pathways. The end result is that the pain response produces activity within the sensory cortex and limbic system. In addition to modulation of the pain signal there is also potential for increased sensitivity of the peripheral nociceptors through repeated exposure to noxious stimuli. Sensitivity has been shown to be further enhanced by a variety of inflammatory mediators associated with tissue injury (Gottschalk and Smith 2001).

MULTIMODAL ANALGESIA

The term multimodal analgesia refers to the implementation of combined strategies to combat pain. Pain management in the 21st century continues to rely heavily on pharmacological approaches, which can be directed at different levels of the pain pathway, i.e., peripheral, spinal, and central, although less obvious non-pharmacological strategies may also play an important role in reducing post-operative pain.

FACTORS CONTRIBUTING TO RISING APPLICATIONS OF LOCAL ANAESTHESIA

Pain Management

Drug related
- Opioids
- NSAIDs
- Local anaesthesia

Non-drug related
- Cryoanalgesia
- TENs
- Acupuncture
- Relaxation

Combined techniques have been well demonstrated to be more effective in the management of post-operative pain than any single strategy. Local anaesthetic techniques have a key role in the management of post-operative pain and this encompasses both the pre- and post-operative phases.

PRE-EMPTIVE ANALGESIA

For many years surgeons have introduced local anaesthetic solutions into surgical wounds at the end of surgery in an attempt to mitigate post-operative pain but this does not produce the same physiological effect as complete neuroaxial blockade prior to the scalpel meeting skin. Crile was the first to describe the value of blocking noxious stimuli from reaching their central target by means of local anaesthetic block. He described this as the so-called "shockless operation" (Crile 1913). This is probably the first description of what today is referred to as pre-emptive analgesia. The concept of pre-emptive analgesia was further evaluated in the 1980s using animal studies and these demonstrated both a decreased stress response to injury and decreased pain in response to injury with the application of pre-emptive analgesic modalities. Surgery under PNB has subsequently been shown to be associated with greater homeostatic stability than the same surgery under general anaesthesia as well as demonstrating a reduced post-surgical analgesic requirement.

Pre-emptive analgesia is however an evolving clinical concept involving the introduction of an analgesic regimen prior to the presence of noxious stimuli with the goal of preventing or reducing the degree of sensitization of the nervous system. Surgery would theoretically be an ideal setting in which to extol the benefits of pre-emptive analgesia because the timing of the noxious stimulus is known. Local anaesthetics are but one of many interventions that might play an important role in the mitigation of post-operative pain.

Pre-emptive analgesia refers to the application of analgesic strategies prior to the procedure aimed at reducing central sensitization to noxious stimuli.

Within this concept of pre-emptive analgesia it has to be remembered that general anaesthesia in itself does not prevent central sensitization. Although patients under general anaesthetic appear to be clinically unresponsive to surgical trauma, the potential for central sensitization exists (Gottschalk and Smith 2001) (Fig. 2.1).

FIGURE 2.1
Pain pathways: potential sites for pre-emptive analgesic strategies.

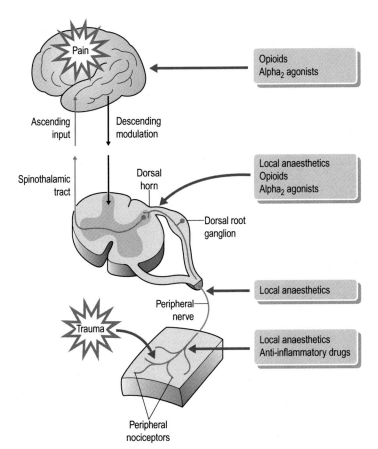

Difficulties arise in determining the efficacy of pre-emptive analgesic strategies because of both variations in the strategies employed and the type of interventions in which they are employed. For example, some studies employ modalities at only one of the potential sites (Pacharinsak et al. 2003). In addition there may be significant variation in the response to pre-emptive analgesic strategies between those that attempt to modulate peripherally and central components of the pain response.

PRE-EMPTIVE ANALGESIC STRATEGIES

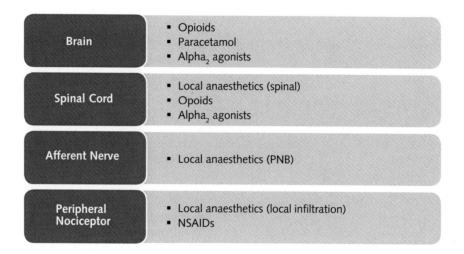

Brain	• Opioids • Paracetamol • Alpha$_2$ agonists
Spinal Cord	• Local anaesthetics (spinal) • Opoids • Alpha$_2$ agonists
Afferent Nerve	• Local anaesthetics (PNB)
Peripheral Nociceptor	• Local anaesthetics (local infiltration) • NSAIDs

The potential benefits of providing adequate post-operative analgesia extend well beyond the immediate patient experience and potential for future sensitization. Reduced post-operative analgesia needs can be correlated with a reduction in medication side-effects, more rapid surgical recovery, and reduced hospital stay. These have huge direct and indirect potential economic benefit.

The evidence for application of local anaesthetic block either by epidural or wound infiltration indicates that greater benefit is gained by pre-operative administration. From a physiological standpoint we do know that the body responds differently when surgery is conducted under general anaesthetic alone as compared to that conducted with the addition of a peripheral nerve block. Kehlet (1989) examined the systemic response to surgical insult noting that PNB was the most effective technique for reducing the endocrine-metabolic response. Put simply a patient undergoing surgery in which the affected body part is under PNB, thereby preventing painful surgical stimuli being transmitted centrally, helps the body maintain its normal metabolic and hormonal status quo.

Literature is replete with evidence demonstrating the beneficial effects of PNB in the field of extremity surgery (Dinley and Dickson 1976; Dahl et al. 1994; Badner et al. 1996; Campbell and Kendrick 1997; Bertini et al. 2001; di Benedetto et al. 2002). The implementation of measures to ensure all patients receive adequate post-operative analgesia will no doubt require compelling evidence that combined strategies are more effective and better collaboration between clinicians involved in the management of the surgical patient.

MANAGEMENT OF ACUTE POST-OPERATIVE PAIN

Despite the very best efforts of the surgical and nursing team some patients will experience excessive post-operative pain and seek assistance. The traditional medical approach is to move up the analgesic ladder introducing stronger analgesics and anti-inflammatories as well as other classes of medicines. Whilst this may appear to be a sensible approach the strategy is fundamentally flawed because:

- Medications modulate pain signals to and within the CNS but do not stop them completely
- Established post-operative pain is less amenable to this therapeutic approach
- Medication side-effects can necessitate patient hospital admission
- PNB can totally obviate the pain signal transmission from periphery to CNS.

When dealing with patients in acute pain following lower limb surgery, administration of a PNB affords almost immediate and total cessation of pain with minimal side effects. Often these patients may be extremely tired and "worn-down" by their pain. Patients frequently defer seeking help until they have taken their full quota of painkillers and can cope no more. Within minutes of administering a PNB they are usually transformed to a more rational state. Whilst these "rescue blocks" are of limited duration, most patients find this additional period of analgesia is sufficient. In any event the PNB can be repeated as necessary before severe breakthrough pain recurs.

It is essential when managing patients in these circumstances to follow a logical management plan. The priority in all cases is to deal with the acute pain by means of a PNB having established there are no contraindications. The next step is to review the surgical site and determine the cause of the pain. Common causes of excessive post-operative pain include haematoma, inadequate initial analgesia, and excessive post-operative mobilization. Finally review the current analgesic plan in place for the patient and decide if this requires any modification. All being well the patient should be able to leave pain free and with strict instructions on what they need to do to minimize a further episode of excessive pain.

1
- **Analgesic Issues**
  - Inadequate initial analgesic plan
  - Failed to commence analgesia until anaesthetic block wore off

2
- **Patient Issues**
  - Anxiety
  - Excessive activity

3
- **Surgical Issues**
  - Tight dressings/casts
  - Haematoma
  - Surgical trauma
  - Peripheral nerve injury

4
- **Medical Issues**
  - Acute Gout

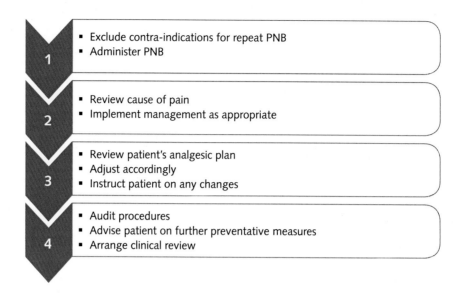

1
- Exclude contra-indications for repeat PNB
- Administer PNB

2
- Review cause of pain
- Implement management as appropriate

3
- Review patient's analgesic plan
- Adjust accordingly
- Instruct patient on any changes

4
- Audit procedures
- Advise patient on further preventative measures
- Arrange clinical review

DIAGNOSTIC INJECTIONS OF THE FOOT AND ANKLE

DIAGNOSTIC INJECTIONS – LOCAL VERSUS DISTAL PATHOLOGY

The foot is a complex anatomical structure subject to a broad range of pathological processes, which may be of intrinsic and extrinsic origin. Local anaesthesia has an important role to play in the diagnosis and management of a number of these pathologies.

Noxious stimuli are conveyed centrally along the afferent nerve fibres to the spinal cord. They may then pass to the brain in the ascending columns of the spinal cord and thus in the case of pain stimuli we become aware of the presence of a painful stimulus and its location. A simplified overview is given in Figure 2.2, which shows the transmission of a stimulus from the foot to the brain.

However, pain thought to arise peripherally can originate centrally. A good example of this is seen in spinal nerve entrapments. A patient may experience symptoms of paraesthesia in the foot as a result of irritation of, for example, the L5 nerve root. In this example the pain is felt in the foot but the pathology is in the spinal cord. Differentiation is important if the patient is to receive the correct treatment. Local anaesthesia blocks the transmission of both afferent and efferent impulses along the nerve by preventing the generation of an action potential. If the injection relieves the symptoms, we can confirm that the underlying pathological process arises distal to the site of injection (Fig 2.3). If, however, symptoms still persist despite anaesthetic block, the problem must arise proximal to the site of the injection (assuming correct injection technique). In this example, the first injection can be placed in the metatarsal interspace. If a Morton's' neuroma is the cause of symptoms, the pain will disappear as the anaesthetic takes effect. If the patient has a tarsal tunnel syndrome, a forefoot injection will fail to resolve the patient's symptoms. A second proximal tibial block could be performed at the ankle. Should this alleviate the symptoms it would point to the pathology being at the level of the ankle.

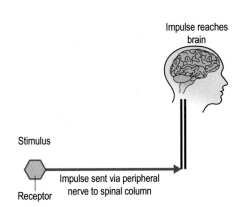

FIGURE 2.2
Schematic of normal afferent input to CNS.

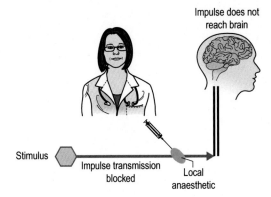

FIGURE 2.3
Schematic of peripheral afferent input blocked by local anaesthetic.

DIAGNOSTIC INJECTIONS – ANAESTHETIZING ADJACENT STRUCTURES

Diagnostic injections can also be used to individually anaesthetize adjacent structures to confirm diagnosis. For example, a patient may present with forefoot pain that presents as either a Morton's neuroma or a lesser metatarsophalangeal joint capsulitis. Unlike the therapeutic technique for administering cortisone outlined in Chapter 12, here we simply wish to block the common digital nerve with local anaesthesia to ascertain the effect. Inject only a small volume of anaesthetic solution so as to avoid inadvertent anaesthesia to surrounding tissues. Review the patient after 15 minutes to see if and how the symptoms have changed. If the pain has gone, it is unlikely that joint pathology is the cause. Conversely, if the presentation is more in keeping with that of capsulitis, the diagnostic block could be performed in the metatarsophalangeal joint.

MANIPULATION UNDER ANAESTHESIA (MUA)

Occasionally, aggressive joint manipulation may be required to increase joint motion. This technique requires a local anaesthetic block for three reasons:

- reduce pain of the manipulation
- diminish muscle tension around joint
- avoid reflex contraction during the manipulation.

Manipulation of the metatarsophalangeal joints may be facilitated by a posterior tibial block supplemented by local infiltration just proximal to the joint. Manipulation of more proximal and larger joints would require more proximal nerve blocks, namely common peroneal and posterior tibial. In view of the loss of protective pain responses, care should be taken when performing joint manipulation under anaesthesia to avoid tearing periarticular soft tissue structures or fracturing osteophytes. Patients should be warned that a moderate degree of discomfort is to be expected once the anaesthetic has worn off.

VENOUS CANNULATION

This procedure involves the insertion of a cannula into a vein in order that access to the venous circulation can be gained, usually for the administration of drugs. The procedure, although readily performed without anaesthesia, can be a source of discomfort to the patient especially where larger bore cannulae are utilized. Any evaluation of patient pain levels during an invasive procedure will be also subject to other influences such as:

- clinical technique
- size of cannula
- psychological profile
- age.

Efforts to overcome this discomfort have been put forward by many medical workers. A well-reported approach involves the topical application of EMLA (eutectic mixture of local anaesthetic) cream at the venepuncture site. The effectiveness of topical local anaesthetic in this setting has been questioned prompting suggestions for more aggressive measures such as subcutaneous local anaesthesia (Selby & Bowles 1995). In their prospective clinical trial, however, EMLA cream was applied for only 5 minutes prior to venous cannulation, insufficient for maximal surface anaesthesia (which requires 30–90 minutes) (Selby and Bowles 1995). It may be that such time scales are impractical in the busy hospital setting. Subcutaneous injection of local anaesthetic provides an effective alternative means of reducing pain associated with venepuncture and is recommended subject to patient suitability. Although both techniques require the clinician to introduce a needle through the skin, infiltration has been found to be significantly less painful than cannulation (Selby & Bowles 1995). Presumably this is due to the smaller gauge needle required for the infiltration coupled with the rapid onset of anaesthesia attainable.

REFERENCES

Akca, O., Melischek, M., Scheck, T., et al., 1999. Postoperative pain and subcutaneous oxygen tension. Lancet 354 (9172), 41–42.

Bachiocco, V., Morselli, A.M., Carli, G., et al., 1993. Self-control expectancy and postsurgical pain: relationships to previous pain, behavior in past pain, familial pain tolerance models, and personality. J. Pain Symptom Manage. 8, 205–214.

Badner, N.H., Bourne, R.B., Rorabeck, C.H., et al., 1996. Intra-articular injection of bupivacaine in knee-replacement operations. Results of use for analgesia and for preemptive blockade. J. Bone Joint Surg. Am. 78, 734–738.

Bertini, L., Borghi, B., Grossi, P., et al., 2001. Continuous peripheral block in foot surgery. Minerva Anestesiol. 67 (9 Suppl. 1), 103–108.

Campbell, W.I., Kendrick, R.W., 1997. Pre-emptive analgesia using local anaesthesia: a study in bilaterally symmetrical surgery. Br. J. Anaesth. 79, 657–659.

Carr, D.B., Goudas, L.C., 1999. Acute pain. Lancet 353 (9169), 2051–2058.

Crile, G.W., 1913. The kinetic theory of shock and its prevention through anoci-association (shockless operation). Lancet 185, 7–16.

Dahl, J.B., Moiniche, S., Kehlet, H., 1994. Wound infiltration with local anaesthetics for postoperative pain relief. Acta. Anaesthesiol. Scand. 38, 7–14.

di Benedetto, P., Casati, A., Bertini, L., et al., 2002. Postoperative analgesia with continuous sciatic nerve block after foot surgery: a prospective, randomized comparison between the popliteal and subgluteal approaches. Anesth. Analg. 94, 996–1000.

Dinley, J., Dickson, R.A., 1976. The control of pain after Keller's operation by the instillation of local anaesthetic before closure. A prospective controlled trial. J. Bone Joint Surg. Br. 58, 356–358.

Gottschalk, A., Smith, D.S., 2001. New concepts in acute pain therapy: preemptive analgesia. Am. Fam. Physician 63, 1979–1984.

Kehlet, H., 1989. The stress response to surgery: release mechanisms and the modifying effect of pain relief. Acta Chir. Scand. Suppl. 550, 22–28.

Kuhn, S., Cooke, K., Collins, M., et al., 1990. Perceptions of pain relief after surgery. BMJ 300, 1687–1690.

Pacharinsak, C., Greene, S.A., Keegan, R.D., et al., 2003. Postoperative analgesia in dogs receiving epidural morphine plus medetomidine. J. Vet. Pharmacol. Ther. 26, 71–77.

Selby, I.R., Bowles, B.J., 1995. Analgesia for venous cannulation: a comparison of EMLA (5 minutes application), lignocaine, ethyl chloride, and nothing. J. R. Soc. Med. 88, 264–267.

BIBLIOGRAPHY AND FURTHER READING

Peng, P.W., Chan, V.W., 1999. Local and regional block in postoperative pain control. Surg. Clin. North Am. 79, 345–370.

Trent, J., 1946. Surgical anesthesia, 1846-1946. J. Hist. Med. Allied Sci. 1, 505–514.

PATIENT SUITABILITY FOR LOCAL ANAESTHETIC

3

Although local anaesthetics are relatively safe drugs and complications associated with their use are few, careful patient assessment remains mandatory as adverse events can and do occur. Assessment of a patient's suitability for peripheral nerve block (PNB) needs to be considered in the context of the block itself and the surgical procedure for which the block is proposed. In this section we will look at the considerations necessary in advance of administering a PNB.

Aspects to Consider Before Administering Peripheral Nerve Block

- Why is a PNB required?
- Driving/machinery
- Social
- Psychological
- Medical

DRIVING

Local anaesthetics and the procedures for which they have been administered may impair a patient's ability to drive or operate machinery safely. Clinicians must use their judgement when advising patients regarding when it is considered safe for them to resume driving. The Driver and Vehicle Licensing Agency (DVLA 2008) offers detailed guidance on this matter. The following is an extract from their current published guidance.

> Drivers do not need to notify DVLA unless the medical conditions likely to affect safe driving persist for longer than 3 months after the date of surgery (but please see Neurological and Cardiovascular Disorders Sections for exceptions). Therefore, licence holders wishing to drive after surgery should establish with their own doctors when it is safe to do so. Any decision regarding returning to driving must take into account several issues. These include recovery from the surgical procedure, recovery from anaesthesia, the distracting effect of pain, impairment due to analgesia (sedation and cognitive impairment), as well as any physical restrictions due to the surgery, underlying condition, or other co-morbid conditions. It is the responsibility of the driver to ensure that he/she is in control of the vehicle at all times and to be able to demonstrate that is so, if stopped by the police. Drivers should check their insurance policy before returning to drive after surgery.

Irrespective of the type of block administered as a minimum it is appropriate to advise against driving until the effects of the anaesthetic block have worn off. A longer period may be appropriate dependent upon the nature and impact of the investigation or procedure performed.

PSYCHOLOGICAL FACTORS

You may have been to the dentist and recall feeling nervous before the appointment. Such feelings are natural, especially where needles are involved. Although procedures performed using local anaesthetics are advantageous, being associated with fewer side-effects than general anaesthetic, their use requires very careful consideration of the patient's psychological status.

Failure to take account of this will place the patient in a situation that will cause unnecessary stress both pre-operatively and intraoperatively. This in itself can have adverse effects on the outcome of a procedure. There are particular difficulties with the use of local anaesthetics with the very young and in those with learning difficulties. It is not possible to give absolute exclusion criteria in these respects since each patient must be considered on an individual basis. It is however always important to discuss with patients what is involved with both the block itself and the subsequent procedure. Both clinician and patient must be satisfied that local anaesthesia is the appropriate choice in each individual case.

In situations where patient anxiety is a concern, it is possible to arrange anxiolytic medication prior to the procedure as an adjunct to the PNB. The provision of pre-operative anxiolytic medication and conscious sedation in combination with PNBs has become more popular as an alternative to general anaesthesia for many procedures and is particularly applicable to lower extremity surgery.

The use of anxiolytic medication does not replace the need for careful patient selection and a good bedside manner. Both are essential when dealing with patients having surgery under local anaesthetic. Particular caution should be exercised with young children (consider both chronological age and maturity) as the combination of sedatives and PNBs are often a poor substitute for general anaesthesia.

> **Considerations Around PNBs and Psychological Suitability**
> - Age
> - Anxiety states
> - Needle phobias
> - Learning disibilities
> - Type of PNB
> - Extent of procedure

MEDICAL SUITABILITY FOR LOCAL ANAESTHETIC

This section will deal with the suitability for the administration of amide-type plain local anaesthetics. It does not include the potential contraindications for anaesthetic agents that incorporate vasoconstrictors. The discussion also assumes that a proper injection technique is employed to prevent accidental intravascular injection, which will impose additional risks.

Summary of Medical Consideration Before Administration of Local Anaesthetic

- Porphyrias
- Epilepsy
- Anaemia
- Anticoagulants
- Neuropathy
- Pregnancy
- Sickle cell
- Methaemaglobinaemia
- Hypersensitivity

EPILEPSY

Epilepsy is a condition in which there are episodes of abnormal patterns of electrical activity of the brain. This results in altered states of behaviour ranging from the apparent day dreaming of petit mal, to the convulsions and seizures of grand mal. High blood levels of local anaesthetics are known to cause convulsions through their action on the CNS. Given this fact, the question arises as to whether these drugs should be given to patients with epilepsy. De Jong discusses the difficulties in answering this question through controlled trials and concludes that local anaesthetics are innocuous in those with seizure disorders because:

- The majority of patients are on controlling medications.
- Known epileptics demonstrated no increased susceptibility to toxicity to "procaine" (Mayer 1924).
- Known epileptics tolerated up to 6 mg/kg of lidocaine without evidence of seizure.
- If resuscitative facilities and anticonvulsant medication are not readily available it would seem prudent to avoid administration of local anaesthetic drugs in poorly controlled epileptics.

ALLERGY

Anaphylaxis is a Type 1 Hypersensitivity reaction. A hypersensitivity reaction is an immunological reaction leading to tissue damage and was first described by Charles Richet in 1902. The term was coined in response to observations made by Richet in which severe, sometimes fatal, reactions occurred in animals on second exposure to foreign protein. Some individuals on contact with antigenic material (e.g., pollen, dust, drugs) produce antibodies of the lgE type that then bind with mast cells. On second exposure to the same antigen, the antigenic material binds with the antibody on the outside of the mast cells, which leads to immediate degranulation of the cell (Fig 3.1). As a result of degranulation, the cell contents are released into local tissue (Table 3.1). The two most important chemicals released that mediate the clinical features of anaphylaxis are histamine and slow-reacting substance of

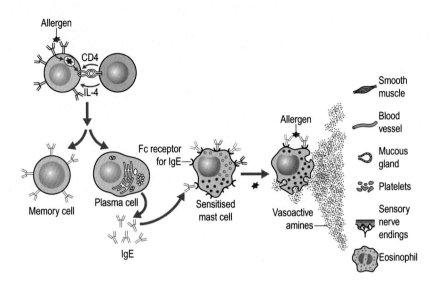

FIGURE 3.1
Allergy. (From http://www-immuno.path.cam.ac.uk)

Table 3.1 Mediators

Primary mediators	
Histamine	Increases vascular permeability Initiates smooth muscle contraction
Serotonin	Increases vascular permeability Initiates smooth muscle contraction
ECF-A	Chemotactic for eosinophil
NCF-A	Chemotactic for neutrophils
Proteases	Connective tissue degradation
Secondary mediators	
Leukotrienes	Increases vascular permeability Initiates smooth muscle contraction
Prostaglandins	Increases vascular permeability Initiates smooth muscle contraction Platelet activation
Bradykinin	Increases vascular permeability Initiates smooth muscle contraction
Cytokines	These induce a wide range of effects including activation of vascular endothelium, eosinophil recruitment and activation

ECF-A, eosinophil chemotactic factor of anaphylaxis; NCF-A, neutrophil chemotactic factor of anaphylaxis.

anaphylaxis (SRS-A). The latter is a product of arachidonic acid metabolism and belongs to a group of substances known as "leukotrienes". This particular substance (SRS-A) is believed to be a strong mediator of respiratory symptoms in a number of conditions, e.g., asthma. SRS-A is a potent constrictor of bronchial smooth muscle and increases vascular permeability and may thus mediate the bronchoconstriction seen in anaphylaxis and laryngeal oedema. The anaphylactic reaction may be local, in which tissue response remains localized to the point of contact between antigen and tissue. Alternatively the reaction may be systemic when inflammatory mediators are released into the circulation. A more generalized response is likely where drugs are administered by injection as in the case of local anaesthetics. The binding of antigen to sensitized mast cells leads to the degranulation of the cell and release of its contents. Local anaesthetics are rare but potent mediators of anaphylaxis. The reported incidence directly attributable to local anaesthetic is less than 1:250 000. A patient with known sensitivity to these drugs is an unsuitable candidate for any local anaesthetic in the podiatric setting. As there is the potential for cross sensitivity between ester and amide drugs selecting a different anaesthetic agent does not guarantee to avoid an anaphylactoid reaction. Unfortunately patients may provide vague accounts of "reactions" to previous local anaesthetic injections. Every attempt should be made to identify patients who have a true history of sensitivity to these drugs. In these circumstances, liaison with an anaesthetist will permit further investigation and safe anaesthetic management.

NEUROPATHY

Peripheral nerve block using local anaesthetics can be complicated by temporary or permanent nerve damage. A variety of mechanisms of injury have been described including direct nerve trauma, toxicity of drug, and neural fluid compression. In view of this potential risk PNBs should be considered carefully in patients with neuropathy. This should include a detailed assessment of motor sensory function.

Subsequent deterioration in neurological status linked temporally to PNB is often directly attributed as the aetiological event. Whilst the processes of consent, detailed record keeping, and meticulous technique are always important, they are especially so when undertaking PNBs in patients with known pre-existing neurological deficit.

SICKLE CELL DISEASE

This is a condition in which there is an abnormality of the haemoglobin. More specifically, this arises because valine is substituted for glutamic acid on the sixth amino acid of the beta chain of haemoglobin (Hb). This haemoglobin is referred to as HbS. The condition is inherited and seen almost exclusively in people of Afro-Caribbean origin. The incidence of homozygotic individuals is approximately 0.3% of blacks in the USA. Homozygotic individuals are said to have sickle cell disease and heterozygotic individuals are said to have sickle cell trait in which there may be few or no symptoms. The consequence of homozygous HbS is as a result of deoxy HbS being much less soluble than deoxy Hb. HbS forms semi-solid rod-like structures within the red blood cells when deoxygenated and thus causes them to sickle. Not only are sickled red blood cells more fragile than ordinary red blood cells, which leads to haemolysis, but they are also less deformable and become trapped in small arterioles and capillaries leading to occlusion and infarction. Individuals who have sickle cell disease should not have tourniquets applied because it will precipitate reduced oxygen tension in the tissues. This is not a contraindication to local anaesthetics as such but would be a contraindication if the anaesthetic was for surgery requiring the use of a tourniquet. Prilocaine hydrochloride however, which can cause methaemoglobinaemia, would be contraindicated in patients with sickle cell disease because at high doses prilocaine can give rise to methaemaglobinaemia, which itself has reduced O_2 carrying capacity.

In patients who have sickle cell disease, it is likely that they will have one or more of the following clinical features:

- severe abdominal pain
- ulcerations
- fever
- arthralgia.

Patients with sickle cell trait do not usually have symptoms and may have a tourniquet applied if it is required for an operation. There are numerous disorders of haemoglobin diseases that may necessitate specialist intervention/advice. If in doubt one should seek the advice of a haematologist or anaesthetist.

ANAEMIA

Except for prilocaine hydrochloride, anaemia does not contraindicate the use of local anaesthetics per se. One does have to contemplate the effects anaemia may have on cardiovascular function and wound healing. Prilocaine is known to cause methaemoglobinaemia if given in high doses (>600 mg) and thus should be avoided in anaemic patients because of the risk of reducing further the oxygen-carrying capacity of blood. Methaemoglobinaemia can be readily treated with intravenous administration of methylene blue.

METHAEMOGLOBINAEMIA

Methaemoglobinaemia can be a side-effect of large doses (>600 mg) of prilocaine. The formation of methaemoglobinaemia is due to a breakdown product of prilocaine, *O*-toludine. *O*-toludine oxidizes haemoglobin to methaemoglobin (met-Hb). Unlike haemoglobin, methaemoglobin is unable to carry oxygen. Sadove (1965) was the first to report this complication of prilocaine administration following the observation of a sudden discoloration of the blood in the operation field after the use of prilocaine (Sadove 1965; Sadove et al. 1965).

The mechanisms for the formation of methaemaglobin are well understood and there appears to be good evidence for a dose–response relationship in the development of methaemoglobinaemia, with noticeable cyanosis occurring with administration of ≥600 mg. What is less well understood is the reason for the significant variation in the amount of methaemoglobin formed by different individuals when exposed to the same dose of prilocaine, i.e., high inter individual variation (Vasters et al. 2006). Vasters and coworkers studied 162 patients undergoing major knee surgery in which a PNB with prilocaine was used. The factors that were associated with increased risk of methaemaglobinaemia following exposure to prilocaine are summarized as follows:

Factors Influential in the Development of Prilocaine Induced Methaemaglobinaemia

Significant risk factor

- Total dose prilocaine
- Younger age > risk met-Hb
- Females
- Use of higher concentrations

Nonsignificant risk factor

- Height
- Weight
- BMI
- PNB site

Maximum levels of met-Hb are usually reached 2–4 hours after prilocaine injection, and return to normal range again after 8–24 hours in most cases. A positive correlation has been shown between the prilocaine dose used for a nerve block and the time until the peak met-Hb. Following a single dose of 300–600 mg prilocaine, met-Hb concentrations in the range of 15% can be detected. Although this is normally considered harmless, in certain circumstances, for example in anaemic patients or in patients with compromised cardiopulmonary function, high levels of met-Hb have the potential to become clinically relevant (Vasters et al. 2006). If clinically necessary methaemoglobinaemia may be treated with methylene blue.

Given the prediction of methaemoglobin levels following administration of prilocaine is subject to significant variation irrespective of total dose administered, when performing PNBs in patients who might be jeopardized by a decreased oxygen transport capacity, clinicians should continue to use lower doses of prilocaine or consider using another local anaesthetic.

When to Consider an Alternative Amide Local Anaesthetic to Prilocaine

- Pregnancy
- Concurrent ester LA
- Breast feeding
- Anaemia
- Known met-Hb

PREGNANCY AND BREAST-FEEDING

The British Medical Association and the Pharmaceutical Society of Great Britain suggest that, because of the risk of harmful effects to the foetus at any time during pregnancy, all drugs should be avoided if possible during the first trimester. Drugs should be prescribed only if the potential benefit outweighs the risk of harm to the foetus. It is worth noting that it is frequently difficult to determine the end of the first trimester. In light of this, it is good advice to avoid administration of local anaesthetics until the patient has had the first scan, which should confirm the stage of foetal development.

With large doses of local anaesthetic neonatal respiratory depression, hypotonia, and bradycardia may occur following paracervical or epidural blocks. There is no guidance on the risks associated with lower limb PNBs. Because of the ability of local anaesthetics to cross the placental barrier, they may be best avoided wherever possible during pregnancy although many pregnant women receive local anaesthetic drugs by way of epidural injections as part of their analgesic management during delivery. If local anaesthetic is to be administered during pregnancy prilocaine hydrochloride should be avoided as foetal haemoglobin is more sensitive to the development of methaemoglobinaemia.

Since no teratogenic effects have been reported in animal studies in doses up to 5 mg/kg of lidocaine, Dollery reports no specific contraindications to the use of lidocaine during pregnancy. Administration of drugs to nursing mothers may affect infants because of the secretion of drug into mother's milk. The possible effects on the infant might include toxicity and theoretically hypersensitivity. Toxicity can develop where the drug enters the mother's milk in sufficient amounts to have a pharmacological effect on the infant. Both lidocaine and bupivacaine are considered safe for use with breast-feeding.

ANAESTHETIC IMPLICATIONS OF MYASTHESIA GRAVIS

Myasthesia gravis (MG) is an autoimmune disease that gives rise to weakness and functional impairment of skeletal muscle. The underlying pathological process is due to a reduction in the number of postsynaptic acetylcholine receptors at the neuromuscular junction. This deficiency impairs the ability of the motor nerve to stimulate the muscle. The condition can be localized to specific muscle groups or generalized throughout the body. In the affected muscle groups there is both diminished power and increased fatigability.

Patients with MG require careful anaesthetic evaluation as their ability to maintain patent airway in the post-operative period may be diminished following a general anaesthetic. Additionally there are a wide range of potential implications associated with anaesthetic drugs such as neuromuscular blocking agents and inhaled anaesthetic agents leading to further respiratory compromise.

With respect to regional anaesthesia the overall risk to the MG patient is less in comparison to general anaesthesia. However potentiation of neuromuscular blocking drugs has been reported. This in theory could lead to increased muscle impairment where local anaesthetic blood levels reach high enough concentrations. Ester-based local anaesthetics are to be avoided in MG patients as they are metabolized by plasma cholinesterases.

PNBs in the lower limb should not present any particular problem in the MG patient so long as due consideration is paid to the overall impact the block may have on a patient's function post injection. For example, an otherwise healthy patient is able to mobilize safely after popliteal PNB despite motor power weakness to the lower leg. In an MG patient mobility may not be feasible due to pre-existing weakness in the limbs.

PNBs IN PATIENTS TAKING ANTICOAGULANTS

Although central neuraxial blockade has been shown to reduce the incidence of thromboembolic events following surgery, many patients either require additional thromboprophylaxis to mitigate their risk further during the perioperative period or thromboprophylaxis for other medical reasons (Table 3.2). Patients with altered coagulation states may present increased risk of injury as a result of PNB. Though this risk is of greatest concern with spinal blocks where devastating vertebral canal haematoma can occur, risks associated with lower limb PNBs should also be considered carefully in advance.

Table 3.2 Anticoagulants

DRUG	COMMON CLINICAL INDICATION	MODE OF ACTION
Aspirin	Thromboprophylaxis in IHD or CVA	Antiplatelet action by inhibiting production of thromboxane A2
Clopidogrel	Acute coronary symptoms	Potent antiplatelet activity. ADP-induced platelet aggregation and platelet–fibrinogen binding are inhibited. Effects are irreversible, platelet function takes 7 days to return to normal
Fondaparinux	Thromboprophylaxis	Synthetic pentasaccharide potent anti-Xa activity. Half life between 17 and 21 h
NSAIDs	Anti-inflammatory	Inhibits platelet function
LMWH	Thromboprophylaxis	Fibrinolytic properties
Warfarin	Thromboprophylaxis,` AF, DVT, PE	Inhibits production of Factors II, VII, IX, X

AF, atrial fibrillation; DVT, deep vein thrombosis; IHD, ischaemic heart disease; LMWH, low molecular weight heparin; PE, pulmonary embolus.

There are no absolute guidelines for the administration of PNBs in patients with altered coagulation states. Each patient should be considered on an individual basis. The risk of haematoma is greatest where needles pass through vascular compartments such as muscle as they are being directed towards nerve. In certain circumstances variation of approach may be sufficient to reduce the risk of haematoma. For example, the popliteal PNB would be best performed via a posterior approach as the lateral approach would necessitate the needle passing through the muscle belly of biceps femoris (short head) whereas the posterior approach does not breach any muscle belly.

PORPHYRIAS

The porphyrias are a group of metabolic disorders due to inborn errors of metabolism of the haem biosynthetic pathway. The metabolic pathway leading to haemoglobin synthesis is complex involving several steps, each of which requires specific enzymatic activity. Each type of porphyria has a characteristic pattern of overproduction and accumulation of haem precursors dependent on the point at which there is enzymatic dysfunction in the haem synthetic pathway.

The porphyrias may be classified according to three characteristics:

1. Major site of abnormal porphyrin production.
2. Acute or nonacute presentation.
3. The pattern of enzymatic deficiency in the haem production.

Haem is synthesized and used by all cells. The two main sites of haem synthesis are erythropoietic and hepatic where haem is incorporated into haemoglobin of the red blood cells and into the hepatic cytochromes. Erythropoietic porphyrias cause extreme skin sensitivity but lack neurological involvement and are not associated with drug-induced crises.

Hepatic porphyrias are associated with abdominal pain, peripheral neuropathy, mental status changes, and are crises often precipitated by "triggering drugs".

Classification of Porphyrias

Hepatic

Hepatic Acute

- Acute intermittent
- Hereditary coproporphyria
- Variegate porphyria
- ALA dehydrase deficiency porphyria

Hepatic Non Acute

- Porphyria cutanea tarda

Erythropoietic

- Uroporphyria
- Protporphyria

Disruption of any part of the biosynthetic pathway can give rise to the clinical condition porphyria. The clinical manifestations may include:

- unexplained peripheral neuropathy
- unexplained abdominal pain
- unexplained psychosis.

The prevalence of this condition varies with geographical location and the specific type of porphyria in question. Most of the carriers of the abnormal gene show no clinical signs of the disorder.

DRUG ADMINISTRATION AND PORPHYRIA

Factors known to precipitate acute porphyric crises include:

- fasting
- dehydration
- infection
- stress
- hormone imbalances
- excess alcohol intake
- administration of certain drugs.

Drug ingestion is a major precipitating factor for acute intermittent porphyrias and a list of known precipitating drugs can be found in current formularies or from the Porphyria Research Unit, Western Infirmary, Glasgow, UK. The main mechanism by which drugs precipitate porphyric crises appears to be a result of decreased haem levels that leads to increased ALA synthetase activity. Included in this list of drugs contraindicated for use in patients with porphyria are some local anaesthetics. These drugs must therefore be avoided in known carriers of the porphyrogenic gene to avoid precipitating an acute attack.

LOCAL ANAESTHETIC DRUGS UNSAFE FOR USE IN ACUTE PORPHYRIAS

Acute porphyria is not an absolute contraindication to PNB though consideration needs to be given to the range of potential precipitating factors and not just the proposed drug administration. The increased stress associated with the perioperative event may serve as a precipitating factor for an acute event.

Of the amide local anaesthetics available both lidocaine and prilocaine are included on this list of unsafe drugs as there is some evidence in animal tissue studies to suggest administration leads to an increase in ALA synthetase activity. Bupivacaine is believed to be safe. A complete list of unsafe drugs may be found in the current edition of the British National Formulary (BNF).

The presence of pre-existing neuropathy requires careful evaluation so as to ensure that any ensuing neurological problems can be differentiated from those already present.

MALIGNANT HYPERPYREXIA

This potentially life-threatening condition can be precipitated by a wide range of drugs, in particular volatile general anaesthetic agents. Local anaesthetics are however believed to be safe and surgery under regional anaesthesia may be a better option for those patients at risk of this complication.

REFERENCES

DVLA, 2008. At a Glance Guide to the Current Medical Standards of Fitness to Drive. http://www.dvla.gov.uk/media/pdf/medical/aagv1.pdf (accessed 19 Jan 2009).

Sadove, M.S., 1965. Clinical experience with Citanest, a new local anesthetic. Acta Anaesthesiol. Scand. Suppl. 16, 271–276.

Sadove, M., Jobgen, E.A., Heller, F.N., et al., 1965. Methemoglobinemia – an effect of a new local anesthetic L-67 (prilocaine). Acta Anaesthesiol. Scand. Suppl. 16, 175–182.

Vasters, F.G., Eberhart, L.H.J., Koch, T., et al., 2006. Risk factors for prilocaine-induced methaemoglobinaemia following peripheral regional anaesthesia. Eur. J. Anaesthesiol. 23, 760–765.

BIBLIOGRAPHY AND FURTHER READING

Checketts, M.R., 2006. Regional anaesthesia in patients taking anticoagulant drugs. Anaesth. Intensive Care Med. 7, 411–413.

Harvey, C.K., 1997. Dilute lidocaine ankle blocks in the diagnosis of sympathetically maintained pain. J. Am. Podiatr. Med. Assoc. 87, 473–477.

Jensen, N.F., Fiddler, D.S., Striepe, V., et al., 1995. Anesthetic considerations in porphyrias. Anesth. Analg. 80, 591–599.

Lew, E., Vloka, J.D., Hadžić, A., 2001. Ropivacaine for peripheral nerve blocks: are there advantages? Tech. Region Anaesth. Pain Manag. 5, 56–59.

CALCULATING MAXIMUM SAFE DOSES

Maximum safe dose (MSD) refers to the amount of drug that can be administered for therapeutic effect with minimum risk of adverse effects. It does not mean that there are no risks from drug administration at or below MSD. In estimating the safe dosage it is important to take into account the rate of absorption, the potency of the drug, and the vascularity of the tissues together with patient factors such as age, weight, and general health.

Within the literature, and in different countries, there is some variation regarding published MSDs for local anaesthetic drugs both in plain solution and in combination with vasoconstrictors. This should infer that there is variation in opinion over the threshold set for a particular drug. We will use two formulas to calculate the MSD to produce an absolute dose in milligrams and a maximum safe volume in millilitres. We will use an approach common in podiatry: note that MSDs per body weight are not available for all drugs. For example, Naropin (ropivacaine hydrochloride) is marketed by AstraZeneca in the UK as a 2 mg/mL (0.2%), 7.5 mg/mL (0.75%), and 10 mg/mL (1.0%) solution. The British National Formulary lists the maximum safe doses as 30–40 mL of a 7.5 mg/mL solution for a major nerve block and 30 mL of a 7.5 mg/mL solution for a field block.

CONSIDERATIONS FOR LOCAL ANAESTHETIC DOSE CALCULATIONS

Patients with high body mass indexes may have increased body fat. Fat is relatively avascular and therefore contributes little to temporary storage of local anaesthetic molecules after absorption. Similarly metabolic capacity is not increased in a linear manner with weight. Although calculations based upon body surface area would provide a more accurate measure of an appropriate dose, body weight is the normal factor against which MSDs are calculated in podiatry. As a guide, in healthy patients a maximal body weight of 70 kg is taken for the calculation of maximum safe dose of local anaesthetic. A person weighing 140 kg does not have a liver mass twice that of someone weighing 70 kg.

When administering local anaesthetics there are two distinct aspects to drug dose.

- maximum dose in any 24 hours
- maximum dose (vol.) to a particular site at one time.

The first relates to the amount of local anaesthetic that may be administered within a 24-hour period before the plasma concentrations are likely to become excessively high so as to risk the onset of toxic effects. Overdose of local anaesthetic is potentially fatal, which is why the amount of drug to be administered should always be carefully calculated. The dosages cited are intended as guidelines only and attention must be paid to the patient's physiological status as this will influence metabolic and excretory capacity. The second consideration with respect to dose is important because administering large volumes of fluid to areas will create pressure within the tissues. Consider the pressure effect of injecting a large volume of fluid around the base of the toe:

- risk of skin necrosis
- compression of vessels and nerves
- risk of toxicity through rapid absorption from a single dose.

Care should be taken to avoid such complications by giving careful thought as to the capacity of local tissues to accommodate the intended volume of local anaesthetic solution. When you administer your local anaesthetic you will give it in the form of a liquid, which will either come in a sealed sterile cartridge, in small multiuse bottles, or in vials. As you give the drug in solution you need to calculate the MSD in volume, usually millilitres (mL). However you will note that the MSDs for different local anaesthetics is given in milligrams (mg) per kilogram of patient body weight (Table 4.1).

Table 4.1 MSD for local anaesthetics

DRUG	BRAND NAME	MSD (PLAIN)
Bupivacaine HCl	Marcain	2 mg/kg
Bupivacaine HCl with adrenaline	Marcain with Adrenaline	As plain soln.
Levobupivacaine HCl	Chirocaine	2 mg/kg
Lidocaine HCl	Xylocaine	3 mg/kg
Lidocaine HCl with adrenaline	Xylocaine with Adrenaline	7 mg/kg
Ropivacaine HCl	Naropin	4.3 mg/kg*
Prilocaine HCl	Citanest	6 mg/kg
Mepivacaine HCl	Scandonest	6 mg/kg

*Not supplied by the manufacturer. Estimated from an MSD of 300 mg.

MSD FOR LOCAL ANAESTHETICS

The values given are essentially a guide as there will be significant variation among patients. In some respects it is the peak plasma concentration that is more important than the actual dose administered.

Factors that increase peak plasma concentration include:

- total drug dose
- rate of absorption
- tissue binding
- plasma protein binding
- rate of metabolism.

The total dose administered is completely under the clinician's control hence the importance of calculating MSDs for patients on an individual basis. Rate of absorption can be influenced by avoidance of intravascular injection and avoidance of sites of high vascularity. The selection of anaesthetic agents combined with vasoconstrictors also aids slowing the speed of systemic absorption.

DOSES WHEN DEALING WITH CONTINUOUS INFUSION OR REPEAT PNB

When prolonged blocks are used either by means of repeat PNBs or continuous infusion the risk of toxicity and peripheral nerve injury needs to be considered. However the cumulative doses safely tolerated often exceed those arrived at by means of calculating MSD against body weight. The following guideline is worthy of note:

> **Ropivacaine**
>
> Cumulative doses of up to 675 mg for surgery and post-operative analgesia administered over 24 hours were well tolerated, as were post-operative continuous epidural infusions. High doses of up to 800 mg per day have been administered with relatively few adverse reactions
>
> (Medical information leaflet 2006 AstraZenica)

CALCULATING SAFE DOSES IN CLINICAL PRACTICE

In the example shown in Table 4.2 there are a few points to consider:

- The calculated maximum safe dose of 24 mL of 0.5% levobupivacaine does not represent a guarantee of an injection free from adverse effects.
- In the event the patient was malnourished, frail, or debilitated in some way one may wish to reduce the total amount of drug administered.
- It does not mean that giving more than 24 mL would lead to an adverse clinical event. These calculations provide a guide and need to be set against the clinical background.

Table 4.2 Calculating local anaesthetic dose

STEP	CALCULATION	EXAMPLE
1	Convert the patient's weight from pounds to kilograms by dividing body weight (lb) by 2.2: $$kg = \frac{body\ weight}{2.2}$$	Mr Smith weighs 132 lb: $$kg = \frac{132}{2.2} = 60\ kg$$
2	Next, calculate the maximum amount of local anaesthetic in mg for this patient: MSD mg = weight (kg) × MSD for drug	We propose to inject Mr Smith with levobupivacaine which has an MSD of 2 mg/kg of body weight. MSD = 60 kg × 2 mg/kg = 120 mg So for this patient we may administer 120 mg of levobupivacaine.
3	The third step is work out what volume of drug this equates to. This will depend on the concentration of the drug administered. MSD (mg) = MSD (mL) × drug % × 10 $$MSD\ (mL) = \frac{MSD\ mg\ for\ patient}{(drug\ \% \times 10)}$$	We decide to administer 0.5% levobupivacaine. The volume to which the MSD of 120 mg equates is thus: 120 mg = MSD (mL) × 0.5 × 10 $$MSD\ (mL) = \frac{120}{5}$$ MSD (mL) = 24 mL

WHAT ABOUT WHEN WE USE TWO DRUGS?

It is often useful to use two different types of local anaesthetic solution in clinical practice. For example, injecting a fast-acting agent initially followed by a local anaesthetic of long duration. The doses for each drug are not additive as the routes of metabolism are essentially similar for all of the amide local anaesthetic agents. The calculation is straightforward and is illustrated in Table 4.3. An alternative method is given in Table 4.4.

Table 4.3 Calculating local anaesthetic dose

STEP	CALCULATION	EXAMPLE
1	Convert the patient's weight from pounds to kilograms if required by dividing body weight by 2.2: $kg = \dfrac{\text{body weight (lb)}}{2.2}$	Mr Smith weighs 154 lb: $Kg = \dfrac{154}{2.2} = 70\ kg$
2	Next calculate the maximum amount of local anaesthetic in mg for this patient MSD mg = body weight × mg/kg for drug	We propose to inject Mr Smith with prilocaine 4% which has an MSD of 6 mg/kg of body weight. MSD 70 kg × 6 mg/kg = 420 mg So for this patient we may administer 420 mg of prilocaine
3	The third step is work out what volume of drug this equates to. This will depend on the concentration of the drug administered: $MSD\ vol. = \dfrac{\text{MSD mg for patient}}{(\text{drug concentration} \times 10)}$	We decide to administer prilocaine for the PNB. The volume to which the MSD of 120 mg equates is thus: $MSD\ vol. = \dfrac{420\ mg}{(4\% \times 10)} = 10.5\,mL$
4	Assume we administer 6 mL of 4% prilocaine to this patient but then wish to follow this with an injection of bupivacaine.	
5	We need to calculate the amount of prilocaine administered with the initial injection: mg = volume × (concentration × 10)	In this example we have administered 6 mL of 4% prilocaine: mg = 6 mL × (4% × 10) = 240 mg of prilocaine has thus been given
6	The next step is to calculate the remaining amount of the first drug that could be administered: Remain MSD = total MSD − mg given	In this case our total initial msd was 420 mg, we have administered 240 mg: Remain MSD = 420 mg − 240 mg = 180 mg
7	The final step is to work out how much body weight the residual possible dose which could be given with drug 1. This is done by dividing the MSD of drug 1 into the amount of remaining MSD: $Equivalent\ body\ wt. = \dfrac{\text{remain MSD mg}}{\text{MSD of drug}}$	In this example we could give a further 180 mg of 4% prilocaine. Prilocaine has an MSD of 6 mg/kg of body weight. To find out what body weight of 180 mg of prilocaine equates to we can simply: $Undosed\ body\ weight = \dfrac{180\ mg}{6\ mg/kg}$ Undosed body weight = 30 kg

Table 4.3—cont'd

STEP	CALCULATION	EXAMPLE
8	It is now a simple calculation to work out the MSD available for drug 2 (bupivacaine) as we effectively work on the basis the patient weighs 30 kg. MSD = 30 kg (body weight) × 2 (MSD bupivacaine) MSD = 60 mg $$\text{Volume} = \frac{60}{(0.5\% \times 10)}$$ Volume = 12 mL Therefore having given our patient an initial dose 6 mL of 4% prilocaine we can administer a further 12 mL of 0.5% bupivacaine Or 24 mL of 0.25% bupivacaine.	

Table 4.4 Calculating local anaesthetic dose

1	An easier way to calculate the maths is to work out the percentage of the MSD that has been given. One may administer 50% of one drug, and 50% of another, or 25%:75%, and so on. For example if you have given a 60 kg patient 4.5 mL of 2% lidocaine, how much 0.5% levobupivacaine could we use? The MSD for this patient is: 60 × 3 = 180 mg 180 mg = volume × 2% × 10 Volume = 180/20 = 9 mL
2	We have given 4.5 mL i.e., half the MSD. We can therefore give half the MSD of levobupivacaine, i.e., Half: 60 × 2 = 120 mg Half: 120 mg = volume × 0.5% × 10 Half: Volume = 120/5 = 24 mL i.e., 12 mL

BIBLIOGRAPHY AND FURTHER READING

Enneking, F.K., 2005. Lower-extremity peripheral nerve blockade: essentials of our current understanding. Reg. Anaesth. Pain Med. 30, 4–35.

Hardie, R.J., Lorimer, D., 2006. Local Anaesthesia in Neale's Disorders of the Foot, Churchill Livingstone, Edinburgh.

Heavner, J.E., 2007. Local anesthetics. Curr. Opin. Anaesthesiol. 20, 336–342.

Joint Formulary Committee, 2008. British National Formulary, fifty sixth ed. British Medical Association and Royal Pharmaceutical Society of Great Britain, London.

Ribotsky, B.M., Berkowitz, K.D., Montague, J.R., 1996. Local anesthetics. Is there an advantage to mixing solutions. J. Am. Podiatr. Med. Assoc. 86, 487–491.

COMPLICATIONS OF PERIPHERAL NERVE BLOCKS

5

Clinicians working with patients should be prepared to deal with common clinical emergencies as the stressful nature of the clinical environment, use of medications, and presence of coexisting medical problems make such events more likely. This is particularly true for those working with more elderly client groups. For those administering PNBs there is the further risk of direct nerve injury associated with block administration, adverse reaction to the local anaesthetic agent, and stress-induced medical complications. This chapter examines the more common complications and examines both preventative and acute management strategies.

Responsibility for the immediate patient care rests with the lead clinician in attendance but efficient management requires a coordinated response by the entire clinical team. Such a response can only be achieved with adequate training for all staff whether they have direct patient contact or not. Training should combine on-site drills aimed at ensuring staff are familiar with procedures as in "fire drills" and more formal training in basic life support. It is necessary to ensure that resuscitation skills are kept up to date; this is especially important as they are seldom required and thus prone to becoming rusty. When they are required, poor technique may make the difference between survival of the casualty or not. Departments should draw up protocols for emergency situations, which identify the roles of individual staff. There should be a regular review of procedures to ensure familiarity with such protocols. More importantly, protocols should be reviewed regularly to ensure compliance with relevant directives. Management of some clinical emergencies requires specialized drugs and equipment.

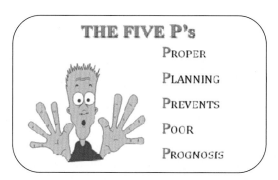

MINIMUM EQUIPMENT RECOMMENDATIONS

The range of drugs and equipment that are necessary when administering PNBs will vary considerably depending on the type of patients being managed and the type of PNBs being undertaken. There is however a minimum level that should be available whenever a PNB is being performed irrespective of how minor the block. The items have been set out in various sections as shown below:

Core
- 2nd staff member
- Policies
- Training records

Equipment
- Telephone
- Oxygen and mask
- Airway
- Cannulae, needles
- Syringes
- Automated external defibrillator
- Suction and tubing

Drugs
- 1:1000 epinephrine × 3
- 100 mg hydrocortisone
- 10 mg chlorpheniramine
- Salbutamol
- Nebulizer

A second person is essential whenever administering drugs as it is not possible to manage a clinical emergency and get the drugs and equipment required ready. Nor is it safe to leave a patient to raise a call to the hospital crash team or ambulance, as this delays intervention time which can be critical to recovery. The training and qualification of the second person will vary according to the nature of the PNBs being administered. As an absolute minimum the person must be trained in their role should they be called upon. The most logical tasks for them to perform would be:

Role of Assistant
- Phone for assistance
- Fetch emergency drugs
- Assist with basic and immediate life support

The decision as to what drugs and equipment are essential is more complex as to some extent this will be influenced by the qualification, training, and competency of the clinicians administering the PNBs. Oxygen is essential; it is simple to administer and can have a dramatic impact on the recovery of the hypoxic patient. Automated defibrillators are becoming simple to use and less expensive nowadays. The probability of successful resuscitation is directly linked to the speed of application and as such it is recommended that one be available in every clinical setting.

TYPES OF COMPLICATIONS

Complications may be considered in four main categories:

Complications of Local Anaesthetics
- Equipment
- Drug
- Clinical emergencies
- Technique

With careful patient selection, appropriate selection of drugs and proper use of the anaesthetic equipment many complications are avoidable. It is however incumbent on the practitioner to ensure he/she is appropriately equipped to deal with these potential problems as and when they occur.

NEEDLE BREAKAGE

As a result of modern manufacturing techniques and single use application, needle breakage is unlikely to ever occur. Sudden patient movement during injection or deliberate bending of the needle during injection will increase the risk of metal fatigue and thus breakage and should therefore be avoided. Needles are weakest at their hub and will break preferentially at this point so it is unadvisable to inject up to this point.

Removal of a broken needle is straightforward as long as the needle is not inserted right up to the level of the hub. This will ensure that should the needle break, a small section will remain visible through the skin. This may then be retrieved with a forceps with little difficulty. In the event that the needle has broken and no fragment can be grasped through the skin, the situation becomes significantly more complicated. In the first instance, the patient needs to be reassured. Keep the patient still to minimize any displacement of the needle and mark the site and direction the needle entered the skin with a permanent marker. Surgical removal under local anaesthetic will be necessary and the needle position will need to be reconfirmed with x-ray where immediate recovery of the needle cannot be facilitated. Provided the clinician is appropriately trained and subject to the availability of the necessary equipment, the foot may be prepped by making a small skin incision directly over the line of the needle beginning at the needle entry point. Using the appropriate technique the needle can be located and removed using a forceps. The skin will need to be closed using an appropriate suture technique. If the facilities and/or expertise are not readily available, the patient will have to be sent to casualty for immediate treatment. In the event the needle is not immediately located it is very likely that intraoperative imaging will be necessary to locate and remove the needle fragment.

NEEDLE STICK INJURY

Gloves offer virtually no protection against needle stick injury but nonsterile gloves should none the less be worn. The principal purpose of wearing gloves is to protect from cross-infection arising from local bleeding after the injection (see DVD). The equipment should be assembled away from the patient on a level, firm platform that does not move. All equipment should be sterile before use and seals checked so that in the event of injury before injection there is no risk of cross-infection to the clinician.

The needle should remain sheathed until immediately before the injection, which is aided by skin tension achieved by the operator's hand(s), which is kept away from the needle at all times. Always wear gloves – not so much to protect yourself from needle stick injury but to protect yourself from blood contact where there is bleeding after the injection(s).

At no time should the operator's hand or any part of it be placed under the needle, for example, under the toe when giving a digital block. Every year clinicians are seen injecting through the patient's toe into their finger or thumb underneath, thus cross-infecting patient and practitioner.

- Ensure equipment is sterile
- Keep fingers clear of needle whilst injecting
- Do not disassemble disposable equipment
- Resheath needles using a single-handed technique
- Never leave equipment lying around
- Never walk around carrying needles and syringes in your hand – always carry in a receiver.

There is no point in resheathing a needle unless you feel it will be required again for the same patient in the immediate future. If this is required resheathing is done single handed by placing the sheath on a tray and introducing the needle into it. On no account should you have syringe and needle in one hand and sheath in the other. This is another ideal way to infect yourself with the patient's blood. As soon as is practicable all used equipment should be disposed of appropriately or taken to be sterilized. Equipment left out is a major hazard to everyone in the clinical environment. Should you be unfortunate enough to suffer a needle stick injury you should take the following action:

- Minimize the risk of further cross-infection
- Encourage copious bleeding of the wound
- Apply a broad-spectrum antiseptic
- Dress the wound
- Contact your own GP or, if available, occupational health department
- Record events in accident book
- If appropriate complete an incident form.

In the event that a patient has been involved you must inform the patient and deal with their wound appropriately. You should take measures to reduce contamination of the patient. In the event of a needle stick injury you should contact your occupational health department immediately for advice.

The National Institute for Health and Clinical Excellence (NICE) (2006) has issued its guidance on the prevention of healthcare-associated infections in primary and community care:

1. Sharps must not be passed directly from hand to hand, and handling should be kept to a minimum.
2. Needles must not be recapped, bent, broken or disassembled before use or disposal.
3. Used sharps must be discarded into a sharps container (conforming to UN3291 and BS 7320 standards) at the point of use by the user.
4. These must not be filled above the mark that indicates that they are full.
5. Containers in public areas must be located in a safe position, and must not be placed on the floor.
6. They must be disposed of by the licensed route in accordance with local policy.
7. Needle safety devices must be used where there are clear indications that they will provide safer systems of working for healthcare personnel.

INTRAVASCULAR INJECTION

Before depositing any anaesthetic it is essential to aspirate to avoid intravascular injection and consequent increased risk of toxicity. Aspiration can be done manually by pulling gently back on the plunger before depositing anaesthetic. With self-aspirating syringes, which use cartridges, aspiration is achieved by pressing the small outer plunger on the syringe, which creates backpressure within the cartridge. If one observes blood entering the syringe it suggests you have the tip of the needle inside a blood vessel. This is not a disastrous event so long as you take the appropriate action before injecting further. When this occurs you have two choices: (1) you may continue through the vessel to the other side; or (2) you may withdraw the needle slightly and redirect it away from the vessel before continuing the injection. The consequences of intravascular injection are:

1. Increased risk of toxicity
2. Damage to vessel wall
3. Arterial bleeding to area with risk of bruising/haematoma formation.

CLINICAL EMERGENCIES

There are a number of distinct phases by which we might approach the management of clinical emergencies (Fig. 5.1). The first and most beneficial is to identify those patients who may be at an increased risk or have greater inherent potential to progress to an untoward clinical event – for example, a known diabetic patient with a history of hypoglycaemic events or a known unstable epileptic patient. Through careful history and physical assessment many patients with such risk factors can be identified in advance. This permits both a greater awareness for the early warning signs and should prompt further review of systems and processes in case such an emergency arises.

Early recognition of a clinical emergency allows prompt intervention, which improves outcomes. The priority will be to manage the patient at greatest medical risk. In the context of dealing with patients receiving PNBs it would be unlikely that more than one patient at any one time would require care. Immediate management should follow best practice guidelines (e.g., Resuscitation Council, UK).

A complete record of any adverse events should be made including any drugs or resuscitative measures employed. In the event of epilepsy the DVLA must be notified by a medical doctor as this will necessitate restriction of driving and certain occupational activities. Most if not all national health service departments will require completion of a "critical incident" form. Depending on the complexity of the emergency faced it may be appropriate for the team members involved to review the events and discuss any issues arising.

We will next examine some of the more common clinical emergencies you may encounter in the clinical situation, some of which have a particular importance to the use of local anaesthetics. Each will be discussed according to the various phases of management described above.

FIGURE 5.1
Strategies in the management
of clinical emergencies.

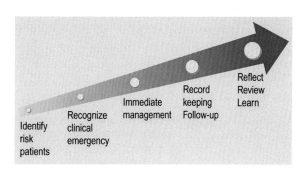

Identify risk patients

Recognize clinical emergency

Immediate management

Record keeping Follow-up

Reflect Review Learn

FAINTING (SYNCOPE)

A faint occurs because of a lack of cerebral perfusion leading to cerebral anoxia. The two commonest mechanisms are:

1. Postural hypotension
2. Stress-induced syncope.

Postural hypotension may occur where the patient rises from a recumbent position quickly leading to a sudden but temporary hypotension. Stress-induced syncope arises because of centrally mediated increased vagal tone. Increased vagal tone may result in reduced cardiac output and syncope. In both instances the event is short lived, with rapid physiological restoration of blood pressure and improved cerebral perfusion.
Clinical features of a faint include:

- Nausea
- Weakness
- Light headedness
- Loss of consciousness
- Initial slow pulse quickly followed by restoration of heart rate.

In the latter situation you may have greater warning that the patient feels light headed/dizzy before they faint. The pulse in the vasovagal faint will be shallow and slow due to the vagal nerve slowing the heart. Management is simple in these situations. The patient is laid flat with legs elevated to help with cerebral perfusion. The vital signs are monitored but the patient should recover within a few minutes and any procedure may continue after the patient indicates they feel well enough. Opening a window or giving the patient oxygen is helpful in these situations. As with all clinical emergencies this must be recorded in the patient's records, which may help the next clinician better prepare the patient and him/herself.

HYPOGLYCAEMIC ATTACK

The patient should be known to you as a diabetic and should have been given appropriate advice with respect to their glycaemic control and diet prior to giving them a local anaesthetic as the stress involved with such procedures may adversely affect their glycaemic control. The patients developing a hypoglycaemic attack may themselves realize that this is happening and request some sugar before symptoms progress. You should seek to recognize this complication early from the following symptoms:

1. Faintness
2. Weakness
3. Tremors
4. Palpitations
5. Hunger
6. Nervousness
7. Confusion
8. Mood changes
9. Loss of consciousness
10. Convulsions.

Provided the patient is conscious you need only give them a drink containing plenty of sugar and they will recover within a few minutes. This may be repeated every 15 minutes if required though it is important to try to avoid a hyperglycaemic attack from developing. If they are unconscious it is unsafe to try to give them glucose orally and such patients must be treated with parenteral drug administration.

The drugs in this case are either:

- 50 mL of 50% glucose IV
- 1 mg glucagon (any route).

If it is not possible to distinguish between a hyperglycaemic attack or hypoglycaemic attack it is advisable to assume hypoglycaemia and manage accordingly as this would not adversely affect the outcome of managing a hyperglycaemic attack should that be the cause of symptoms. Many diabetic patients will be aware that their blood sugar is too low and notice the "early warning signs" themselves. There are however a number of circumstances in which these early warning signs themselves may be less apparent:

- Patients receiving insulin
- Patients taking beta-blockers
- Symptoms may only develop at lower blood glucose levels in those with tight glucose control.

Most clinics involved with performing surgery should be equipped with instruments for assessing capillary blood glucose (glucometers), which are sufficiently quick to be of practical value in the management of such a situation.

DIABETIC KETOACIDOSIS

This situation is less common than diabetic hypoglycaemic attacks but is still a clinical emergency when it arises. Features of hyperglycaemia include:

- Polyuria
- Thirst or hunger
- Air hunger
- Acetone (pear-drop) odour to breath
- Nausea and vomiting.

If in doubt a rapid evaluation of the patient's blood glucose should be performed if reagent strips or a glucometer is available. If there is difficulty in distinguishing between a hypogly-caemic and hyperglycaemic attack it is best to treat as if it is a hypoglycaemic attack and assess the patient's immediate response. Failure to respond indicates the initial assessment is incorrect. In such situations the patients can be given insulin but will require hospitalization.

ANGINA

This is not a direct complication of the local anaesthetic agent itself but may be precipitated by the increased levels of stress during the perioperative period leading to increased sympathetic activity and release of catecholamines, which increases the demands on the heart and thus may precipitate an attack of angina. A history of stable angina does not contraindicate the use of local anaesthetics although it should alert the astute clinician to increased importance of patient reassurance and the increased possibility of this as a clinical emergency. Patients with a history of unstable angina will not make suitable candidates for surgery under local anaesthesia unless medical support is immediately available. The features of an angina attack are:

- Known history of cardiovascular disease (sometimes)
- Varied discomfort from vague to intense pain related to stress/anxiety/physical activity
- Pain located in sternum or chest – may radiate to left arm
- Heart rate and blood pressure increase during attack
- Usually of short duration unless progresses to a myocardial infarction (MI)
- Relieved by glyceryl trinitrate spray/tablet.

The patient will probably be aware that he or she is experiencing an angina attack and should have appropriate medication with them. This should be administered immediately. If the attack does not subside within a few minutes then the patient should be given medical attention by calling an ambulance or crash team if one is available.

MYOCARDIAL INFARCTION

A myocardial infarction will require urgent medical assistance because early management with appropriate drugs has been clinically proved to reduce morbidity and mortality following such attacks. The clinical features of a myocardial infarction are:

- Known history of cardiovascular disease (sometimes)
- Pain similar but more severe than that of angina
- Patient restless but highly anxious
- Patient may appear cyanosed
- Pain not relieved by glyceryl trinitrate.

Immediate management requires making sure that the patient is comfortable and giving reassurance to try to reduce anxiety as far as is practicable. The patient's vital signs should be monitored and appropriate action be taken should resuscitation become necessary. If available and so long as the patient is conscious one half a standard 300 mg aspirin tablet should be administered as soon as possible. Administration of aspirin in this situation has been shown to improve the prognosis following myocardial infarction. The patient should be removed to hospital as soon as possible afterwards for follow-up evaluation.

TOXICITY

Toxicity is generally considered to result from overdose or from intravascular injection giving rise to rapid rises in plasma concentrations of the local anaesthetic agent. Normally peak plasma concentrations develop approximately 15–20 minutes following injection but this will vary and is dependent on such things as site of injection and the vascularity of the injection site. It is because the local anaesthetic agent is able to cross the blood–brain barrier one can observe toxicity as initial central nervous system excitation, which may progress to eventual central nervous system depression and coma. Initial signs and symptoms may include some or all of the following:

Features of Toxicity
- Perioral numbness/tingling
- Restlessness
- Excitement/nervousness
- Dizziness
- Tinnitus
- Blurred vision
- Muscle twitching/tremors
- Convulsions
- Coma
- Death

Factors Impacting on Plasma Concentrations
- Total dose
- Rate of absorption
- Vascularity of tissues
- Vasoactivity of drug
- Pattern of distribution
- Rate of metabolism

Convulsions may develop, which will require energetic management with the administration of intravenous anticonvulsants by a medical practitioner. Although toxicity is normally first manifested by the signs indicated in the box, convulsions can be the first signs of toxicity and it is therefore incumbent on the practitioner using local anaesthetics to ensure that resuscitation equipment is available. Recognition of the early features of toxicity is aided by slow injection technique and a good patient rapport during the injection period so that early changes in the patient's status may be noted and appropriate action taken. This excitatory phase may be followed by central nervous system depression with drowsiness, respiratory failure, coma, and, if untreated, death. There may also be simultaneous cardiovascular effects with depression of cardiac activity and peripheral vasodilatation, which will require monitoring and early management with correct positioning of the patient. Although toxicity is more likely if the maximum recommended safe doses are exceeded, adverse reactions can occur at doses below the recommended safe limits and may be a consequence of rapid absorption from intravascular injection or injection into sites of high vascularity. Management of toxicity requires early recognition so that injection may be terminated and the patient's vital signs restored.

Lipid rescue

Toxicity associated with PNBs is a potentially fatal clinical event and may occur more frequently than most clinicians realize. It is likely that mild toxicity goes underreported and that the increasing application of PNBs may contribute to a rise in toxic sequelae, although newer local anaesthetic agents with broader therapeutic indices may help counter this.

Incidence of toxicity

In a review of complications of 100 000 brachial plexus blocks (Auroy et al. 1997) there were 200 cases of toxicity and three deaths (Table 5.1). In a large Japanese study (Irita et al. 2005), the incidence of toxicity was 1.17 per 100 000 cases of regional anaesthesia. Until recently there was no effective antidote to severe local anaesthetic toxicity. Intralipid was originally proposed by Dr Weinberg, an anaesthetist at the University of Chicago. His work was initiated by a chance observation made during a series of experiments testing whether a lipid infusion would increase arrhythmias during bupivacaine toxicity. More recently animal studies of bupivacaine-induced cardiac arrest have suggested a role for intravenous administration of Intralipid in counteracting the local anaesthetic toxicity.

Table 5.1 Incidence of toxicity

UK 2000–4	BRACHIAL PLEXUS BLOCKS	FATALITY	INCIDENCE
• 3 deaths as a direct result of intravenous bupivacaine administration	• Incidence of toxicity: 200/100000	• 0.023/ 100000	• Large Japanese study: the incidence was 1.17/100000 (Kawashima 2006)

How Intralipid works is unknown though it has been postulated that Intralipid, which is a lipid emulsion, may simply absorb the local anaesthetic or, alternatively, it introduces a large supply of fatty acids, which may act as an energy source for the depleted myocardium in cardiac arrest (Malachy & Maclennan 2007). Despite the fact that no human studies have been undertaken, Intralipid has been recommended for unresponsive cardiac arrest resulting from local anaesthetic toxicity (Picard & Meek 2006; Malachy & Maclennan 2007). There have been several human case reports of successful resuscitation when using Intralipid, one of which involved bupivacaine-related cardiac arrest, and another involved ropivacaine-related asystole (Litz et al. 2006; Rosenblatt et al. 2006). Intralipid has also been successful in reversing pure central nervous system toxicity and, in addition to asystole, other abnormal heart rhythms such as superventricular tachycardia may respond to the intervention?

Despite the lack of controlled trials, which are unlikely to be undertaken given the ethical implications, the Association of Anaesthetists of Great Britain & Ireland has recently produced guidelines for the management of severe local anaesthetic toxicity (AAGBI 2007). In addition to the life-saving measures described by the Resuscitation Council, the Association of Anaesthetists recommends the confirmation or establishment of IV access, and in the event of cardiac arrest cardiopulmonary bypass should be considered as should lipid emulsion treatment (Intralipid).

During an arrest the Association recommends an initial 100 mL bolus of 20% Intralipid 1.5 mL/kg over 1 minute followed by continued cardiopulmonary resuscitation (CPR). An intravenous infusion should then be started with 20% Intralipid 0.25 mL/kg over 1 minute at a rate of 400 mL over 20 minutes. If no return of circulation is noted two further 100-mL bolus injections can be given at 5-minute intervals. If these fail a further bolus can be given: 400 mL of 0.5 mL/kg over 10 minutes. The guidelines state that if this fails infusion should be continued until return of circulation. Further guidance and support on the use of Intralipid is also freely available to clinicians online via the Lipid Rescue website (Weinberg 2007).

Intralipid summary

1. Treatment of life-threatening local anaesthetic overdose.
2. Toxicity is a potentially fatal consequence of local anaesthetic administration.
3. Administration of Intralipid has been shown to be effective when all other measures to resuscitate have failed.

Immediate Management of Acute Toxicity

- Stop injecting the LA
- Call for help
- Maintain the airway
- Give 100% oxygen
- Confirm or establish intravenous access
- Control seizures
- Access cardiovascular status throughout
- Start cardiopulmonary resuscitation (CPR) using standard protocols
- Manage arrhythmias using the same protocols
- Prolonged resuscitation may be necessary
- Consider the use of cardiopulmonary bypass if available
- Consider treatment with lipid emulsion

Management of Severe Toxicity

- Follow ALS/ILS protocol
- Gain IV access asap
- Unresponsive cardiac arrest?
- Consider Intralipid for confirmed LA toxicity

Intralipid Practical Aspects

Treatment of cardiac arrest with lipid emulsion:

- Give an intravenous bolus injection of Intralipid 20% 1.5 mL/kg over 1 min
- Continue CPR
- Start an intravenous infusion of Intralipid 20% at 0.25 mL/kg over 20 min
- Repeat the bolus injection twice at 5 min intervals if an adequate circulation has not been restored
- After another 5 min, increase the rate to 0.5 mL/kg if an adequate circulation has not been restored given at a rate of 400 mL over 10 min
- Continue infusion until a stable and adequate circulation has been restored
- To be administered only after failure of standard resuscitation attempts

Intralipid Adverse Reactions

Catheter-related sepsis:

- Thrombophlebitis
- 1% Dyspnea
- 1% Cyanosis

Allergic Reactions

Delayed reactions:

- Jaundice/hepatomegaly
- Contains aluminium, which may reach toxic levels

SUMMARY

- Severe toxicity is a rare event.
- Post injection; patients should be monitored by surgical and nursing staff for signs of toxicity.
- Urgent 100% oxygen application is essential to minimize acidosis.
- Ensure resuscitation equipment is readily available.
- Gain IV access early.
- In case of unresponsive cardiac arrest consider IV Intralipid.

NERVE INJURY RELATED TO PERIPHERAL NERVE BLOCKS

Peripheral nerve blocks have become well established in medical and surgical practice. The very fact these techniques require placement of a needle in close proximity to a peripheral nerve or nerve plexus affords the potential for nerve injury. Concern over iatrogenic neurological damage may be heightened in today's climate of ever increasing medical litigation. The situation is compounded by the fact that any nerve injury following peripheral nerve block is often automatically attributed to the block with little consideration for other potential causes. In fact many medical claims are settled even though a PNB remains unproven as the cause of any subsequent neurological complication.

When considering the various aetiologies of nerve injury in the context of PNBs the reader should also keep in mind the fact that neurological deficit following PNB may be temporally related but unrelated to the actual injection itself. Table 5.2 summarizes some of the possible causes of nerve injury. We will now look in more detail at the issues surrounding PNBs and neurological complications (Table 5.2).

Table 5.2 Aetiology of neurological damage associated with PNBs

BLOCK RELATED	BLOCK UNRELATED
Normal anaesthetic effect	Tourniquet injury
Intraneural injection	Surgical insult
Needle trauma	Cast complication
Haematoma	Insensate injury

INCIDENCE OF NERVE INJURY ASSOCIATED WITH PNBs

It is difficult to accurately establish the true incidence of nerve injury following PNBs, not least because of the potential for underreporting of more minor or transient complications. Published data suggest an incidence of between 0.2% and 0.4% though this mainly relates to brachial plexus rather than lower limb blocks. Furthermore no studies compare the relative risks of PNBs in the conscious, sedated, and anaesthetized patient. What is clear however is that serious and long-lasting neurological complications associated with PNBs are rare but can and do occur (Table 5.3).

Table 5.3 Data on PNB-associated Injury

Auroy et al. (1997) Prospective evaluation of complications associated with regional anaesthetic techniques in nearly 104 000 blocks over a 5-month period in France. Of the 34 patients noted to have neurological complications following regional anaesthetic block (including PNBs) complete recovery was seen in 19 of these patients within 3 months	Neurological complications were seen in only 34 of the patients with the highest incidence associated with spinal anaesthesia though the following complications occurred in association with PNBs: • 3 cardiac arrests • 1 death • 16 seizures • 4 neurological injury
Auroy et al. (1997) Follow-up study using self-reported questionnaires assessing for serious complications over a 10-month period. Total of 50 223 PNBs	1 cardiac arrest 2 acute respiratory failure 12 peripheral neuropathy

CLINICAL IMPACT OF NEUROLOGICAL INJURY ASSOCIATED WITH PNBs

Whilst various studies have confirmed the risk of neurological sequelae associated with PNBs is very low, it is important to remember that any "risk analysis" must consider both the frequency and magnitude of any potential complication (Auroy et al. 1997). Foot drop as a consequence of common peroneal nerve injury might be a rare event but would be catastrophic to the patient.

PERIPHERAL NERVE BLOCKS IN THE ANAESTHETIZED PATIENT

There would appear to be some division of opinion over the appropriateness of performing peripheral nerve blocks in the anaesthetized patient. Those who argue against the safety of such techniques do so mainly on the premise that the conscious patient will be able to forewarn of impending intraneural injection thus avoiding injury whereas in the anaesthetized patient any protective mechanism is lost. It is difficult to see how this assumption stands up to much scrutiny for a number of reasons:

- Many of the patients in whom neurological injury has followed PNB did not report pain during their injection.
- Damage associated with intraneural injection may well occur immediately, especially with intrafascicular injection, thus the damage is already done.
- A degree of pain is anticipated with the administration of any PNBs. Coupled with individual variation in pain threshold, interpretation of patient feedback is difficult.

PNBs in children are seldom a success without recourse to sedation or general anaesthetic. The value of combining general anaesthetic with PNB in regard to reduced post-operative pain as compared to same surgery without the addition of PNB is not to be underestimated. For this reason it is widely accepted that administering PNBs in anaesthetized children is totally acceptable for the reduced post-operative pain. It is not difficult to apply a similar argument for adults where the addition of a good PNB after induction in combination with good analgesic regimens can obviate excessive post-operative pain.

BASIC ANATOMY OF PERIPHERAL NERVES

To appreciate the simplified mechanisms of nerve injury presented in this section we will need to briefly review the normal anatomy of the peripheral nerve (Fig. 5.2). This will allow us to appreciate better the various mechanisms of nerve injury.

FIGURE 5.2
Normal anatomy of the peripheral nerve.

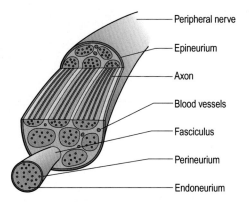

Peripheral nerve

Epineurium

Axon

Blood vessels

Fasciculus

Perineurium

Endoneurium

Peripheral nerves are the electrical wiring system of the body that conduct electrical impulses. The nerves can be likened to a typical electrical cable, which is made up of many finer strands contained within a sheath. The outermost covering is the "epineurium"; this is a tough fibrous sheath that protects the entire peripheral nerve bundle. Within this are contained many individual bundles of axons grouped together (fascicles). The fascicles are themselves surrounded by a layer of tissue referred to as the "perineurium".

CLASSIFICATION OF ACUTE NERVE INJURY

Sunderland has classified acute nerve injury into three subgroups, which reflect the degree of nerve damage and thus the ultimate chance of nerve recovery:

Neuropraxia
- Results from a mild amount of trauma
- Results in failure of a nerve conduction across the damaged segment
- Complete recovery can be expected in the absence of further damage or other physiological insufficiency

Axontmesis
- Disruption to the axon but the endoneurium remains intact. Functional recovery requires regeneration of the axon, which occurs slowly (1–3 mm/day)
- Slow recovery may also be complicated by incomplete restoration of nerve function

Neurotmosis
- Most severe form of nerve injury with complete disruption of the nerve through either "crush" or "transaction" injury
- There is both axonal and endoneural damage
- The prognosis is poor and permanent neurological deficit is to be expected

Neuropraxia represents the mildest form of injury with temporary disruption of nerve function due to mild trauma. In the absence of continued insult and absence of physiological insufficiency complete recovery can be expected. Axonotmesis occurs where there is a greater degree of neuronal insult with physical disruption to the axon but maintenance of the endoneurium. Recovery requires regeneration of the damaged segment, which is a slow process (1–3 mm per day). Crush or laceration of the nerve gives rise to the most severe form of injury, neurotmesis, with both endoneural and axonal damage. This type of injury has a poor prognosis and permanent functional impairment can be expected.

NERVE INJURY IN PNBs

> **Nerve Injury in PNBs**
>
> **Mechanical**
> - Laceration
> - Stretch
> - Compression
>
> **Vascular**
> - Acute ischaemia
> - Chronic ischaemia
>
> **Chemical**
> - Exposure to neurotoxins
>
> **Other**
> - Accidental injury

There are a number of mechanisms that may result in injury to the peripheral nerves that may be associated with PNBs. As discussed earlier it is necessary to consider those that give rise to direct nerve injury during performance of the PNB (PNB-related) and also those that are unrelated to the PNB per se.

Mechanical injury

Laceration can occur as a result of needle trauma during the PNB. Larger-diameter (small-gauge) needles, repeated needle passes, and needle tip design are all relevant to the risk of direct nerve trauma. Intraneural injection may give rise to nerve injury by both direct and indirect trauma. Laceration of the nerve by the cutting needle tip leads to obvious damage. The risk of damage is known to be greatest if the needle enters the fascicular bundles and is less likely to result in injury if it merely pierces the sheath but spares the fascicles. Deliberate or indeed accidental intraneural injection is to be avoided wherever possible. However, even with excellent technique and the application of nerve stimulators, it is not always possible to avoid accidental intraneural needle placement. Methodical and slow needle technique will contribute to reducing the risk and is to be encouraged in all clinicians performing PNBs. Locating nerves by eliciting paraesthesia with the needle tip has been advocated by many as an excellent method of nerve localization (Horlocker et al. 1997; Horlocker & Wedel 2000). Although there remains some controversy as to the inevitability of neurological complications where needle paraesthesia is seen, common sense would seem to direct us to abandon this technique where alternative and potentially safer alternatives exist. Whilst other techniques may result in accidental "needle paraesthesia" this is quite different from deliberately setting out to create it when we know there is an increased potential for intraneural injection.

A nerve stimulator (Fig. 5.3) provides a practical method by which the relationship between the needle tip and peripheral nerve can be determined. Whilst there are no absolute figures for stimulator output and needle tip to nerve distance, nerve stimulators provide the clinician with a safer alternative technique for nerve localization and are associated with great PNB efficacy compared with "blind" injection techniques.

Figure 5.3
Typical nerve stimulator.

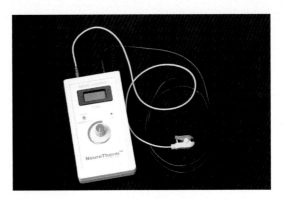

Resistance to injection

Intrafascicular injection is associated with the greatest risk of damage to the peripheral nerve due to the damage to the perineurium and disruption of the delicate fascicular anatomy. Intrafascicular injections are also associated with higher injection pressures and this should be borne in mind by the clinician when administering PNBs. Unusually high resistance to injection should alert the clinician to inadvertent intraneural injection. Injections associated with pressures greater than 20 psi have been associated with clinically detectable neurological deficits.

Intraneural injection is more likely to result in unusually rapid onset of anaesthesia as would be expected as the axons are exposed to very high concentrations of local anaesthetic solution, which has only a short diffusion distance to its target site of action. Whilst initially appealing to the clinician the very real risk of neurological damage as a result of intraneural damage should encourage the clinician to develop techniques to deposit local anaesthetic solution as close as possible to the desired peripheral nerve without entering it.

Stretch

Excessive stretch applied to the nerve can disrupt normal function leading to injury. Care should be exercised when positioning patients who have had PNBs and therefore lost the normal protective reflexes.

Compression

PNBs are typically administered in the surgical setting during which time the patient is subject to other interventions, which are a potential cause of nerve injury. The application of a pneumatic tourniquet, which allows better surgical visualization through maintenance of a bloodless field, mandates high cuff pressures (Fig. 5.4).

FIGURE 5.4
Ankle tourniquet.

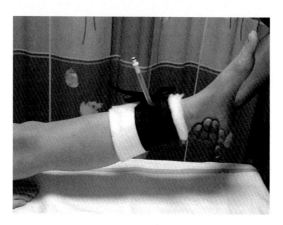

Thigh tourniquet pressures in the order of 200–300 mmHg are typical. At the ankle the peripheral nerves are superficial and cross bony structures rendering them vulnerable to compression injury in the insensate foot. Peripheral nerves are also at risk of injury from the resultant ischaemia.

VASCULAR INJURY

All living tissues have certain metabolic requirements for which an adequate vascular supply is essential. Nerves are no different and vascular compromise leads to neural ischaemia and disruption of normal neuronal metabolic pathways. If deprived long enough permanent nerve dysfunction ensues. Peripheral nerves have a dual blood supply consisting of intrinsic (endoneural) vessels and extrinsic (epineural) vessels. The epineural vessels are susceptible to adrenergic stimuli and thus addition of vasoconstrictors may potentially contribute to neuronal ischaemia (Niemi 2005). The delicate intraneural vasculature has very low capillary pressures and thus any extrinsic forces may be sufficient to overcome capillary pressure thus leading to temporary ischaemia. Intraneural injection of anaesthetic solution will result in increased hydrostatic pressure with even small volumes of anaesthetic solutions. Larger volumes administered externally to the nerve can result in occlusion, especially where the nerve is contained within a fibro-osseous tunnel or other space-limited environment. Consider the patient with intermittent claudication who is unable to walk more than 100 yards without developing severe calf pain as a result of metabolic demand of the calf muscle exceeding the supply due to ischaemia. Peripheral nerves are no different; inadequate blood supply leads to metabolic stress. Vascular compromise may be the result of acute ischaemia or haemorrhage.

Acute ischaemia

This may arise from extrinsic causes, e.g., compression of arteries due to planned tourniquet inflation or compression of blood vessels due to malplacement of the insensate limb during a period of anaesthesia.

Haemorrhage

Haemorrhage around peripheral nerves is potentially a cause of compression leading to both direct and indirect nerve injury. This risk may be increased in those patients receiving concomitant anticoagulant therapy. In the initial phases of peripheral nerve ischaemia there is spontaneous depolarization of axons within the peripheral nerve and generation of spontaneous activity, which is perceived by the patient as "paraesthesia". We have all experienced the feeling of "pins and needles" at one time or another down the leg after sitting awkwardly for a period of time. The impact of ischaemia on nerves is time dependent. Where ischaemia lasts less than 2 hours full nerve recovery can be expected. Ischaemia for prolonged periods (>2 hours), however, is associated with more serious structural changes within the nerve. After reperfusion intraneural oedema develops along with degeneration of axons. There then follows a period of regeneration which may take several weeks. Recovery may be incomplete if ischaemia was prolonged.

INJURY TO THE INSENSATE LIMB

The insensate extremity is also "at risk" as normal protective reflexes are impaired for the duration of the anaesthetic block. There is a risk to the ill-informed patient of exposing the limb to injury without realizing. Simple malpositioning of the limb leading to compression of tissues against chairs, beds, etc. needs to be avoided. Diminished protective reflexes and motor power increase the risk of falls and mandate good patient compliance in addition to detailed record keeping of instructions given.

The application of casts post-operatively is frequently necessary to protect the operative site. At the same time most foot surgeons would employ the use of long-acting local anaesthetics as part of their strategy. The application of a cast to an anaesthetized limb poses a dilemma to the clinician. Inadvertent excessive cast pressure would go unnoticed and risks pressure ulceration. However use of short-acting local anaesthetics will deprive the patient of adequate pain relief. Even the strongest of analgesics fails to compete with a good regional block in managing post-operative pain. Failure to protect the limb with a cast risks serious damage to the operation site. Whilst each case should be considered individually the author experience has been that adequate post-operative analgesia followed by protection of the surgical site takes precedence. To this end the author is happy to employ a well-padded back-slab to the lower limb in the immediate post-operative period whilst the limb remains anaesthetized.

CHEMICAL INJURY: NEUROTOXIC SUBSTANCES

Local anaesthetics are frequently described as having a fully reversible action with no deleterious effects to peripheral nerves. However local anaesthetics do produce a variety of cytotoxic effects including inhibition of cell growth and cell death. These effects appear to be proportional to the degree of exposure (both time and concentration). The presence of pre-existing neurological complications (neuropathy, nerve injury) may increase the risk of nerve injury from local anaesthetic toxicity at clinical doses. Repeat injection or the use of indwelling catheters for the provision of continuous anaesthetic infusion increases nerve exposure. For obvious reasons our understanding of the neurotoxic effects of local anaesthetics has largely come from animal studies and observation data following unexpected events in patients receiving these drugs. It would be difficult to see many "ethics committees" allowing human subjects to be exposed to toxic doses of local anaesthetic solution for perceived scientific benefit.

Sakura and coworkers (1995) investigated whether local anaesthetic neurotoxicity was associated with sodium channel blockade or whether other mechanisms were responsible. They compared the effects of intrathecally administered lidocaine, bupivacaine, and tetrodotoxin (TTX), the latter a highly selective sodium channel blocker. Interestingly they were able to demonstrate that neurotoxicity does not result from sodium channel blockade. This then poses the question of what mechanisms may be at play in the development of neurotoxicity and raises the possibility of identifying drugs that are equally effective as local anaesthetics but which have reduced neurotoxicity.

There is some evidence that the observed neurotoxicity of local anaesthetics may relate to mitochondrial degradation. Local anaesthetics lead to depolarization of plasma membranes and this effect is seen in mitochondria, the cell's energy producers. Depolarization of mitochondria leads to reduced ATP production, the cellular energy currency. Loss of ATP leads to a slowing/cessation of energy-dependent processes. Loss of ATP also impairs axonal transport mechanisms. In addition at high concentrations local anaesthetics have been shown to form "micelles", which may act as a detergent disrupting the normal phospholipid cell membrane.

NEEDLE DESIGN

The hypodermic needle allows penetration of the skin and delivery of local anaesthetic to the desired anatomical location. The selection of needles for individual blocks is discussed in greater detail in Chapter 8. In the context of nerve injury however it is worth a brief discussion regarding needle tip design. There are principally two types of needle, short bevel (30–45° tip angle) and long bevel (12–15°). Selander and colleagues suggested penetration of the nerve fascicle was less likely with a short bevel needle. However more recent work by Rice and McMahon (1993) demonstrated that penetration of the nerve fascicle with long bevel needles (12–27°) resulted in less damage than that of short bevel needles. It is suggested that a sharp needle results in a clean cut and less blunt trauma. Nerve penetration with needles during PNB is probably more common than first realized and carries real risk of nerve injury. It is likely that the combination of nerve penetration by the needle followed by injection of local anaesthetic carries a greater risk of injury.

REDUCING THE RISK OF INJURY FOLLOWING PNB

Though individual clinical judgement must remain central to the administration of PNBs some general guidelines may prove beneficial in minimizing complications or at the very least substantiating "best practice" in the event complications do occur.

ASEPTIC TECHNIQUE

Hands of healthcare workers are the main route of transmission of micro-organisms of nosocomial infections. However, compliance with hand hygiene procedures is still insufficient. Rubbing hands with alcohol-based solutions in order to decontaminate hands instead of handwashing, as proposed in new recommendations, is one way of solving the problem (Simon 2004). Although the bactericidal effect of skin disinfectants (povidone iodine and chlorhexidine) peaks at 2 minutes (O'Grady 2002) it is common to leave skin cleansing as the last step before skin infiltration, which does not leave adequate time for disinfectants to be effective. However, in a review of the literature no cases of infection attributable to PNB were identified. Other authors have questioned the value of preinjection skin antisepsis claiming there is no proven clinical benefit (Metz 1973; Lieffers and Mokkink 2002). This issue should, however, be viewed from a risk–cost benefit standpoint. The measures required to reduce cross-infection have tiny cost implications. The consequences of infection from PNB are potentially very costly to both patient and healthcare provider. Furthermore, in the course of medicolegal work, the authors have dealt with a claim for negligence where a patient developed septic arthritis the day after receiving an ankle block anaesthetic; no other intervention was given. The claimant's lawyers made a case on the basis of *res ipsa loquitur* (Latin: the thing speaks for itself). It refers to situations where it is assumed that a person's injury was caused by the negligent action of another party because the accident was the sort that would not occur unless someone was negligent.

For these reasons we would advocate that all patients receiving a peripheral nerve block should be managed along the following lines:

- Use disposable equipment only
- Multidose vials should be changed daily
- Drawing up needles should be used and fresh needles utilized for injections
- Operator should wear nonsterile gloves
- Injection sites should be cleansed with an appropriate skin disinfectant.

Perhaps more importantly these "best practice" measures must be part of a written clinical protocol so that in the event of a complication it can be demonstrated that appropriate clinical standards were in place.

NEEDLE SELECTION

As a rule of thumb the smallest gauge needle should be picked that is suitable for the PNB to be undertaken. Recommendations are given under each of the techniques described. In addition to considering the diameter of the needle, an appropriate length needle should be selected. Excessively long needles pose an increased risk of inadvertent tissue damage and inappropriately short needles may fail to deliver anaesthetic solution to the desired anatomical location or necessitate an increased number of injection points.

ANATOMICAL LOCALIZATION

PNBs of the lower limb can be challenging at the best of times. Undertaking such blocks where local anatomy is obscured because of increased body fat or altered as a result of previous surgery or congenital deformity adds to the difficulties. The clinician undertaking blocks faced with such additional challenges needs to adapt his/her technique accordingly. The first goal of any PNB is to determine the needle entry point such that it will then allow easy localization of the peripheral nerve. Identifying key anatomical landmarks is an essential first step to this process.

Identify and mark key osseous landmarks but acknowledge any alteration due to previous surgery or congenital abnormality.

Give further consideration to the location of major tendon insertions by having the patient tense the respective muscles against resistance so you are then able to mark these structures accurately. If the patient is to have their block whilst anaesthetized this needs to be done in advance.

Finally the use of a Doppler machine will allow accurate localization of arteries and veins. The value of Doppler should not be underestimated because even when local anatomy has been distorted or is obscured by body fat there is nearly always consistency of major neurovascular bundles.

SPEED OF NEEDLE POSITIONING

During the course of PNBs, needle advancement should be controlled and slow. Rapid movement of a needle through tissues serves no useful purpose and increases the risk of inadvertent injury to both clinician and patient. Using a logical and controlled technique the clinician is much more likely to avoid accidental intraneural injection as well as increasing the chance of nerve localization when using a nerve stimulator. Remember that the electrical output from a nerve stimulator occurs in pulses, the speed of which is determined by the output frequency of the unit (Hz). So a machine set with an output of 2 Hz in practical terms delivers pulses of electrical current twice a second. When in close enough proximity to the peripheral nerve this leads to depolarization and an action potential. Clinically we see the relevant muscle contraction. Rapid advancement of the needle during nerve localization can mean the impulses output of the nerve stimulator misses the point of closest proximity.

SPEED OF INJECTION

There are many reasons why anaesthetic solution should be administered in small incremental doses. Rapid infusion of solution leads to a build up of pressure locally within the tissues, which is painful in itself. Slow incremental injection allows the anaesthetic fluid to be distributed more readily, minimizing pain of injection. Perhaps more importantly inadvertent intravascular injection can and does occur even with negative aspiration. Rapid injection of high volumes of anaesthetic solution deprives the clinician of the opportunity to recognize the early signs of toxicity and avoid further dose administration. Once administered the drug cannot be removed so it is better to administer in an incremental manner allowing a short interval between each bolus.

> **Safe Injection Cycle for PNBs in Lower Limb**
> - Confirm needle placement
> - Administer 3–4 mL solution
> - Monitor for signs of toxicity

INJECTION PRESSURE/RESISTANCE

This is perhaps one of the most subjective of all aspects of the injection. We know from the previous discussion that intraneural injection is associated with unusually high resistance to injection (injection pressure) and that it can be associated with serious neurological sequelae. The best that can be conveyed is that the clinician should endeavour to get a "feel" for what is usual with regard to expected injection resistance for a range of PNBs.

This "feel" has to take into account the equipment being used and the anatomical site of the injection being administered. Consider that using very fine gauge needles will be associated with a feeling of higher resistance compared with larger-diameter needles. This is amplified where larger syringes are attached to fine gauge needles.

EXCESSIVE INJECTION PAIN

For most people being injected is painful. Despite various attempts to develop "pain-free" systems, the introduction of a needle through intact sensate skin evokes a pain response, which varies from person to person. With due regard to the individual patient and technique being employed, clinicians should try to identify those patients who report "excessive pain on injection". Whilst it is not possible to define what constitutes excessive pain, with experience clinicians will be able to differentiate the usual injection discomfort and mild paraesthesia that can be associated with injections. Severe pain on injection points to intraneural injection with consequent risk of nerve injury. In this circumstance the injection should be stopped and consideration given to aborting the procedure to allow time for proper neurological evaluation.

REPEAT BLOCKS/TOP-UP ANAESTHETIC

Those who claim 100% success with their PNBs are clearly more gifted than the rest of us. Failure of PNBs is to be anticipated and whilst we all strive to make this number as close to zero as possible it is inevitable. This is especially true for those of us who perform surgical procedures without any adjunctive sedation where there is little tolerance for partial block failure. The question thus arises as to how to manage those patients in whom a PNB has failed either partially or totally. Whilst the risk of nerve injury would intuitively be proportional to the number of injections administered (all else being equal) one must balance this with the consequence to the patient of not proceeding with "rescue" anaesthesia. It would seem perfectly reasonable to make every effort to achieve a successful PNB even where this requires repeated injections. This does require that the clinician pays due regard to both the rescue technique and total dose administered. Discussion with the patient should be documented in regard to proceeding with further injections or departure from the original anaesthetic plan (i.e., moving from a planned local anaesthetic procedure to general anaesthetic).

DIAGNOSIS AND MANAGEMENT OF PERIPHERAL NERVE INJURY ASSOCIATED WITH PNB

Recognition of peripheral nerve injury following PNBs is often delayed because of the anaesthetic action itself masking pain or motor loss. The surgical event itself may also compound the difficulties of early recognition by virtue of the fact that patients may mistake neurogenic pain with post-operative pain. The addition of casts, splints, and pain medications all adds to the potential delay in recognition.

The spectrum of pain from neurological insult arising from PNB is broad both in terms of severity and also temporally. Symptoms may range from minor tingling and numbness through to complete motor sensory loss.

SPECTRUM OF CLINICAL FEATURES ASSOCIATED WITH PERIPHERAL NERVE INJURY (FIG. 5.5)

FIGURE 5.5
Spectrum of clinical features associated with peripheral nerve injury.

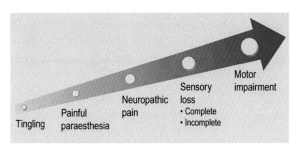

Patients in whom neurological injury is suspected require careful and thorough assessment to determine the level of the suspected nerve injury and the impact. Evaluation of sensory and motor function will assist the clinician in determining both the level of the nerve injury and the severity. The prognosis for patients with mild paraesthesia is good, with most people showing full recovery within 3 months. Where more serious injury is suspected, neurological opinion should be sought at the earliest opportunity so that more detailed investigations may be considered. These may include:

- Electrophysiological testing/nerve conduction
- High-resolution ultrasound
- MRI scan.

The goal is to fully determine the exact location of the nerve insult and where possible to assess the severity. High-definition ultrasound is able to provide detailed imaging of peripheral nerves such that it is possible to visualize morphological changes in the nerve itself. Unlike EMG testing, ultrasound is painless. Compared with MRI, ultrasound is faster and cheaper to perform though it does require radiologists who have specific expertise in assessing these types of pathologies.

RECORD KEEPING AND PERIPHERAL NERVE BLOCKS

Clinical records never look as bad as when as the clinician are required to rely on them to justify your actions at the behest of a prelitigation claim or complaint. There is rarely a time when the author asked to review a case where the clinicians involved content with the quality of their records. Sadly when it comes to dealing with these matters it is largely the contemporaneous notes that are relied upon in evidence. More than this though, the notes provide a rich source of data, which can allow the clinician to reflect upon the outcome of their intervention(s).

With any general anaesthetic administered the anaesthetist would be expected to complete a hospital "anaesthetic chart". From experience it appears there is a lack of standardized charting for the administration of PNBs. Admittedly the incidence of complications arising from a general anaesthetic may be greater than those associated with PNBs, however the consequences of complications remain potentially serious. For this reason we would recommend a minimum data set is maintained against each PNB administered (Table 5.4). The simplest way to achieve this is by the adoption of a standard anaesthetic sheet. This can be tailored to an individual department's needs where required so as to ensure minimal complexity yet demonstrate adherence to minimum practice guidelines.

Table 5.4 Recommended data set for all PNBs

BASIC DATA	DRUGS	TECHNIQUE	OTHER
Name Address Date of birth ID number Medical suitability for proposed PNB Consent	Calculation of MSD Drug name Drug volume/concentration	Skin antisepsis Block type Patient position Stimulator current on injection	Top-up block(s) Excessive injection pain Adverse reactions Postinjection advice

LOCAL ANAESTHETICS AND EPINEPHRINE

Epinephrine has been added to local anaesthetics for over a century. It has two principal benefits arising principally from its vasoconstrictive properties:

- Reduced peak plasma concentrations
- Enhanced local anaesthetic duration.

These beneficial effects are seen with both central neuroaxial blocks as well as PNBs. The local vasoconstriction at the site of injection is believed to reduce blood flow and thus delay anaesthetic clearance (Niemi 2005). This assumption is well supported by experimental data, which demonstrate reduced peak plasma concentrations when epinephrine is added to local anaesthetic agents (Myers & Heckman 1989; Liu et al. 1995; Bernards & Kopacz 1999). The increase in duration of local anaesthetic action is less in long-acting local anaesthetic drugs as compared to short-acting agents.

When administered intravenously epinephrine has both α- and β-adrenergic receptor agonist activity. The effect is dose-dependent when given IV. Stimulation of α1 and α2 receptors leads to vasoconstriction of blood vessels. Arteries contain mainly α1 receptors whereas veins contain mainly α2 receptors. Stimulation of beta receptors in the heart (β1 + β2), skeletal muscle blood vessels (β2), pulmonary vessels, and superior mesenteric and splenic arteries leads to marked physiological changes. Cardiac output is increased as a result of increased contractility of the heart (stroke volume) plus an increase in heart rate. At the same time there is reduced peripheral resistance due to vasodilatation.

Cardiac output = stroke volume × heart rate

Blood pressure = cardiac output × total peripheral resistance

The net physiological effect will depend on which of the two systems dominates, which is in turn determined by the plasma concentration of epinephrine. The relevance in clinical practice is twofold: first the addition of epinephrine has implications for the potential risks associated with PNBs due to potential increased cardiac stress; second many patients claiming allergy to local anaesthetics, if not nearly all of them, actually refer to a sudden and short-lived cardiovascular effect of epinephrine when receiving local anaesthetic injection at the dentist. This is usually determined by the nature of the symptoms (palpitations, sweating, and increased pulse rate) which is of a very short duration (the half-life of epinephrine is <3 minutes). In addition to the beneficial effects associated with the vasoconstrictive properties, epinephrine may also exert a positive pharmacodynamic analgesic effect through its α2 effect. It is possible that adrenoreceptors may modify potassium channels in the axons of peripheral nerves potentiating the effect of sodium channel blockers (i.e., local anaesthetics).

REFERENCES

AAGBI, 2007. Guidelines for the Management of Severe Local Anaesthetic Toxicity, The Association of Anaesthetists of Great Britain & Ireland, London.

Auroy, Y., Narchi, P., Messiah, A., et al., 1997. Serious complications related to regional anesthesia: results of a prospective survey in France. Anesthesiology 87, 479–486.

Bernards, C.M., Kopacz, D.J., 1999. Effect of epinephrine on lidocaine clearance in vivo: a microdialysis study in humans. Anesthesiology 91, 962–968.

Horlocker, T.T., Wedel, D.J., 2000. Neurologic complications of spinal and epidural anesthesia. Reg. Anesth. Pain Med. 25, 83–98.

Horlocker, T.T., McGregor, D.G., Matsushige, D.K., et al., 1997. Neurologic complications of 603 consecutive continuous spinal anesthetics using macrocatheter and microcatheter techniques. Perioperative Outcomes Group. Anesth. Analg. 84, 1063–1070.

Irita, K., Kawashima, Y., Morita, Y., et al., 2005. Critical incidents during regional anesthesia in Japanese Society of Anesthesiologists-Certified Training Hospitals: an analysis of responses to the annual survey conducted between 1999 and 2002 by the Japanese Society of Anesthesiologists. Mausi Japan J. Anesthesiol. 54, 440–449.

Lieffers, M.A., Mokkink, H.G., 2002. Disinfection of the skin prior to injections does not influence the incidence of infections; a literature study. Ned. Tijdschr. Geneeskd. 146, 765–767.

Litz, R., Popp, M., Stehr, N., Koch, T., 2006. Successful resuscitation of a patient with ropivacaine-induced asystole after axillary plexus block using lipid infusion. Anaesthesia 61, 800–801.

Liu, S., Carpenter, R.L., Chiu, A.A., et al., 1995. Epinephrine prolongs duration of subcutaneous infiltration of local anesthesia in a dose-related manner. Correlation with magnitude of vasoconstriction.
Reg. Anesth. 20, 378–384.

Malachy, C., Maclennan, K., 2007. Local anaesthetic agents. Anaesth. Intensive Care Med. 8, 159–162.

Metz, H., 1973. Skin disinfection before injections not necessary? Med. Klin. 68, 128–129.

Myers, R.R., Heckman, H.M., 1989. Effects of local anesthesia on nerve blood flow: studies using lidocaine with and without epinephrine. Anesthesiology 71, 757–762.

National Institute for Clinical Excellence, 2006. Clinical Guideline 2: Infection Control. http://www.nice.org.uk

Niemi, G., 2005. Advantages and disadvantages of adrenaline in regional anaesthesia. Best Pract Res Clin. Anaesthesiol 19 (2), 229–245.

O'Grady, N.P., Alexander, M., Dellinger, E.P., et al., 2002. Healthcare Infection Control Practices Advisory Committee: Guidelines for the prevention of intravascular catheter-related infections. Infect. Control Hosp. Epidemiol. 23, 759–769.

Picard, J., Meek, T., 2006. Lipid emulsion to treat overdose of local anaesthetic: the gift of the glob. Editorial Anaesthesia 61, 107–109.

Rice, A.S.C., McMahon, S.B., 1993. Peripheral nerve injury caused by injection needles. Br. J. Anaesth. 71, 324–325.

Rosenblatt, M.A., et al., 2006. Successful use of a 20% lipid emulsion to resuscitate a patient after a presumed bupivacaine-related cardiac arrest. Anesthesiology 105, 217–218.

Sakura, A., Bollen, A.W., Ciriales, R., Drasner, K., 1995. Local anesthetic neurotoxicity does not result from blockade of voltage-gated sodium channels. Anesth. Analg. 81, 338–346.

Simon, A.C., 2004. Hand hygiene, the crusade of the infection control specialist. Alcohol-based handrub: the solution! Acta Clin. Belg. 59 (4), 189–193.

Weinberg, G., 2007. Lipid Rescue: Resuscitation for Cardiac Toxicity 2007. Available at: http://www.lipidrescue.org

BIBLIOGRAPHY AND FURTHER READING

Birt, D., Thomas, B., Wilson, I., 1999. Resuscitation from cardiac arrest. Update in Anaesthesia 10, 6. Available at: http://www.nda.ox.ac.uk/wfsa/

Brull, S.J., 2008. Lipid emulsion for the treatment of local anesthetic toxicity: patient safety implications. Anesth. Analg. 106, 1337–1339.

DiFazio, C.A., 1981. Local anesthetics: action, metabolism, and toxicity. Otolaryngol. Clin. North Am. 14, 515–519.

Glinert, R.J., Zachary, C.B., 1991. Local anesthetic allergy. Its recognition and avoidance. J. Dermatol. Surg. Oncol. 17, 491–496.

Groban, L., Butterworth, J., 2003. Lipid reversal of bupivacaine toxicity: has the silver bullet been identified? Reg. Anesth. Pain Med. 28, 167–169.

Horlocker, T.T., 2001. Neurologic complications of neuraxial and peripheral blockade. Can. J. Anesth. 48 (6), R1–R8.

Litz, R.J., Roessel, T., Heller, A.R., Stehr, S.N., 2008. Reversal of central nervous system and cardiac toxicity after local anesthetic intoxication by lipid emulsion injection. Anesth. Analg.106: 1575–1577.

Phillips, J.F., Yates, A.B., Deshazo, R.D., 2007. Approach to patients with suspected hypersensitivity to local anesthetics. Am. J. Med. Sci. 334, 190–196.

Rowlingson, J.C., 2008. Lipid rescue: a step forward in patient safety? Likely so! Anesth. Analg. 106, 1333–1336.

Scott, D.B., 1981. Toxicity caused by local anaesthetic drugs. Br. J. Anaesth. 53, 553–554.

Weinberg, G., Garcia-Amaro, M., Cwik, M., et al., 1998. Pretreatment or resuscitation with a lipid infusion shifts the dose-response to bupivacaine-induced asystole in rats. Anesthesiology 88, 1071–1075.

Weinberg, G., Ripper, R., Feinstein, D., Hoffman, W., 2003. Lipid emulsion infusion rescues dogs from bupivacaine-induced cardiac toxicity. Reg. Anesth. Pain Med. 28, 198–202.

NERVE STIMULATORS

6

Nerves conduct action potentials either from the periphery centrally (afferent) or in the opposite direction (efferent). These action potentials are generated when a stimulus of an appropriate intensity is applied leading to depolarization of the nerve membrane. A nerve stimulator is an artificial means of generating an action potential. The idea was first developed by Von Perthes in 1912 but there was little clinical application until the 1980s when interest in regional anaesthesia surfaced and the need to locate peripheral nerves without direct visualization became apparent. The value of the nerve stimulator is simply that it allows the clinician to attain close needle to nerve proximity thus increasing the chance of successful peripheral nerve block. In addition to improving the overall success rates of PNBs the use of a nerve stimulator has been shown to greatly decrease the anaesthetic dose required for successful block (Fig. 6.1).

FIGURE 6.1 Comparison of nerve blocks with and without nerve stimulator

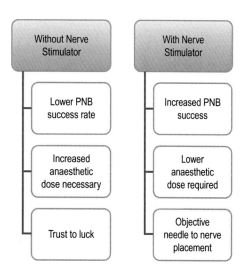

HOW DOES A NERVE STIMULATOR WORK?

These devices work by supplying electrons to depolarize a nerve (Fig. 6.2). The number of electrons supplied per stimulus equals the current output of the nerve stimulator. The greater the current output the greater the potential for the nearby nerve to become depolarized thus evoking contraction of the muscle supplied by that particular nerve. As the needle to nerve distance decreases depolarization will occur at progressively (though in a nonlinear manner) lower current outputs. This is the basic principle by which the nerve stimulator is useful in localization of peripheral nerves.

FIGURE 6.2
Concept of nerve stimulator function.

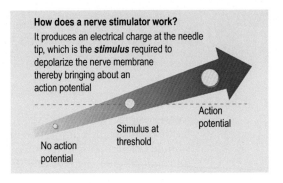

How does a nerve stimulator work?
It produces an electrical charge at the needle tip, which is the **stimulus** required to depolarize the nerve membrane thereby bringing about an action potential

No action potential

Stimulus at threshold

Action potential

KEY COMPONENTS OF A NERVE STIMULATOR

Whilst there are many models available to choose from there are some fundamental elements to consider when selecting a nerve stimulator (Table 6.1).

Table 6.1 Features of ideal nerve stimulator

Large digital display	A large display indicating the current output and battery status is useful in clinical practice especially for those blocks which require the anaesthetist to adopt somewhat awkward positions
Battery indicator	It can be distressing for the clinician and the patient when a battery failure goes unnoticed and proves to be responsible for the lack of success in locating the peripheral nerve
Constant current output	As the resistance between needle tip and electrode changes the voltage output must increase or decrease if the current output is to remain the same. Some of the older nerve stimulators were of a fixed voltage output so when the resistance increased the effective current output decreased ($V = I \times R$). Most modern nerve stimulators are able to maintain a constant current during normal use by varying the voltage delivered
Short pulse duration	Short pulse duration ensures that nerve stimulator output preferentially stimulates only A-alpha fibres (motor fibres) thus minimizing pain during nerve localization
Frequency output of 1–2 HZ	The optimum pulse frequency is between 1 and 2 Hz. Frequencies of greater than 2 Hz lead to muscle fasciculation. Lower frequencies may result in the needle being advanced before delivery of a further impulse thus risking close needle to nerve relationship being missed by the operator
Control of current intensity	All nerve stimulators must be able to deliver a variable current output, which is readily controlled electronically. The type of controller depends on the unit design. Considerations should include the ease of use and the degree of output control offered by the unit
Malfunction indicator	All units must include automated warning systems in the event of electrical malfunction

PLACEMENT OF ELECTRODES

The outside of a "resting" nerve has a net positive charge due to the imbalance of sodium, potassium, and chloride ions between the inside and outside of the nerve membrane. It is "polarized". Adding negative electrons to the outside of the axon (via a nerve stimulator) will neutralize this charge, i.e., induce depolarization and thus evoke an action potential. The indifferent electrode (ECG tab) may be placed at any point on the limb to be blocked. The over-riding requirement is good skin/electrode contact.

TYPES OF NERVE STIMULATOR

There are a wide variety of nerve stimulators available. It is useful to understand the major characteristics that can impact on their clinical application.

CHANGING RESISTANCE

The impedance between the electrodes and the skin is not constant. If the electrodes dry out or come loose from the skin their resistance will increase. There are two ways a nerve stimulator can respond to this change: with a constant voltage or a constant current. Ohm's law applies to electrical circuits; it states that the current passing through a conductor between two points is directly proportional to the potential difference (i.e., voltage drop or voltage) across the two points, and inversely proportional to the resistance between them. The mathematical equation that describes this relationship is:

$$I = \frac{V}{R}$$

where V = voltage, I = current, and R = resistance. As the impedance (resistance) increases, for the current to remain constant the voltage must increase. This current delivered in the context of nerve stimulators is effectively the number of electrons delivered at the needle tip and therefore directly related to the chance of depolarization.

CONSTANT VOLTAGE NERVE STIMULATORS

Constant voltage nerve stimulators are relatively easy and cheap to make. Unfortunately if the voltage remains constant when resistance increases then the current must decrease. As a result the nerve may not be completely stimulated. The muscle contraction will then be depressed. The anaesthetist will falsely think that the neuromuscular blocking drug is still working. This can be dangerous if the patient moves during a delicate phase of surgery. Some constant voltage nerve stimulators will display the current actually delivered and will alarm if it falls below some predefined threshold.

CONSTANT CURRENT NERVE STIMULATORS

Constant current nerve stimulators are the safest but also the most expensive to build. As the resistance between the needle and skin electrode increases voltage is automatically increased so as to maintain the desired current output. There is however a limit to how high the nerve stimulator can raise the voltage and remain safe for clinical applications. At this point the stimulator should give an audible and visual alarm that the stimulating current has not been reached.

WHY DON'T NERVE STIMULATORS CAUSE PATIENTS PAIN DURING THEIR USE?

To understand why nerve stimulators used in PNBs preferentially stimulate motor fibre response we must first look at two important neurophysiological terms:

- Rheobase – minimum current required to evoke an action potential over unlimited pulse duration
- Chronaxie – duration of the current required to evoke an action potential with a stimulus twice that of the Rheobase.

We can therefore define the susceptibility of a nerve fibre by its Chronaxie. Nerve stimulators are engineered in such a way as to take advantage of this, thereby avoiding unnecessary stimulation of nerve fibres other than those responsible for motor activity (Table 6.2).

Table 6.2 Susceptibility of nerve fibre type and stimulus duration

FIBRE TYPE	DURATION OF STIMULUS TO EVOKE ACTION POTENTIAL
A-alpha	50–100 μs
A-delta	170 μs
C	400 μs

SENSITIVITY OF MOTOR ACTIVITY TO CURRENT OUTPUT

Although most authors would agree that prior to injection a motor response to a current output close to 0.5 mA is desirable, this is not always possible. Perlas and coworkers confirmed needle placement in brachial plexus blocks using high-definition ultrasound and were able to show that in roughly 75% of patients motor response was evident at a current of 0.5 mA; the remainder of their group required an output of up to 1 mA in order to elicit a motor response (Fig. 6.3).

FIGURE 6.3
Sensitivity of motor response.
(Data from Perlas et al. 2006.)

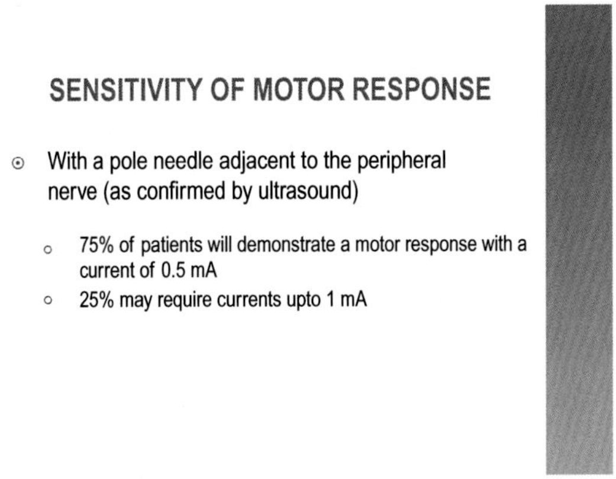

SENSITIVITY OF MOTOR RESPONSE

⊙ With a pole needle adjacent to the peripheral nerve (as confirmed by ultrasound)

    ○ 75% of patients will demonstrate a motor response with a current of 0.5 mA
    ○ 25% may require currents upto 1 mA

INSULATED NEEDLES

We have seen that the mechanism by which a nerve stimulator works in clinical practice is via the delivery of electrons at the needle tip. In order to ensure that this electrical output remains as focused as possible the needle length is insulated with only the very tip exposed (Fig. 6.4). This design ensures that the field of electrical output remains focused in a smaller point, thus increasing the accuracy of the injection.

FIGURE 6.4
Insulated and noninsulated
needles.

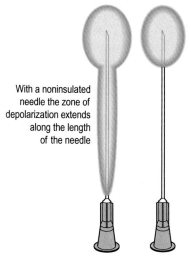

Insulated needle
has zone of
depolarization
localized to the
needle tip

With a noninsulated
needle the zone of
depolarization extends
along the length
of the needle

PRACTICAL STEPS WHEN USING A NERVE STIMULATOR (FIG. 6.5)

FIGURE 6.5
Practical steps when using a
nerve stimulator.

Prepare the equipment in advance checking battery especially.
Needles, gloves, drugs and skin electrode are essential

Prepare the patient by explaining the procedure. Position
them correctly to allow the PNB to proceed comfortably for
you and the patient. Clean the skin

Mark the needle entry point according to the particular block
technique. Position skin electrode ensuring good contact.
Connect the equipment and ensure the unit is set to "locate"

Locate the needle through the skin and set the unit to an
output of 2–3 mA.
Advance the needle slowly in desired direction watching for
the desired motor activity

When desired motor activity is observed gradually
reduce output to determine maximal motor response
with mimimial current output. This determines the
best needle position for the PNB

With motor response seen at an output of between
0.5–1 mA inject local anaesthetic slowly and
incrementally observing the patient's status
throughout

These devices are straightforward to use but familiarity with the equipment before facing the patient is always helpful. Patients must be monitored carefully following all PNBs and given strict instructions on mobilization. This is especially relevant to popliteal blocks where substantial motor weakness to the leg risks injury.

Warning – Injections should not proceed if motor activity is observed at currents of 2 mA or less as this suggests intrafascicular injection.

BIBLIOGRAPHY AND FURTHER READING

Bollini, C.A., Cacheiro, F., 2006. Peripheral nerve stimulation. Tech. Region Anesth. Pain Manag. 10, 79–88.

Chelly, J.E., Greger, J., Gebhard, R., et al., 2002. Training of residents in peripheral nerve blocks during anesthesiology residency. J. Clin. Anesth. 14, 584–588.

De Andrés, J., Alonso-Iñigo, J.M., Blanch, X.S., Reina, M.A., 2005. Nerve stimulation in regional anesthesia: theory and practice. Best Pract. Res. Clin. Anaesthesiol. 19, 153–174.

Doty, R., Sukhani, R., Kendall, M.C., et al., 2006. Evaluation of a proximal site and the use of nerve-stimulator-guided needle placement for posterior tibial nerve block. Anesth. Analg. 103, 1300–1305.

Fanelli, G., Casati, A., Garancini, P., Torri, G., 1999. Study group on regional anaesthesia. Nerve stimulator and multiple injection technique for upper and lower limb blockade: failure rate, patient acceptance and neurological complications. Anesth. Analg. 88, 847–852.

Visan, A., Vloka, J.D., Koenigsamen, J., Hadžić, A., 2002. Peripheral nerve stimulators technology. Tech. Region Anesth. Pain Manag. 6, 155–157.

THE BASICS 7

As with many clinical interventions there is often more than one way of achieving the desired goal. Nerve blocks are no different and the literature is replete with variations of techniques. Having administered many thousand lower limb blocks the author hope to provide the reader with a sensible and reliable approach, after all, it is all well and good pursuing a technique that uses slightly less anaesthetic agent but if your success rate is diminished as a consequence the benefit is lost.

The information presented is deliberately standardized for ease of reference but this does not imply that it is necessary to adhere strictly to volume or drug volumes indicated. These are a guide only and due regard should be given to the physical status of each patient. Before we look at the individual techniques however there are a few other important aspects worthy of consideration that relate to the administration of a peripheral nerve block.

WARMING THE LOCAL ANAESTHETIC SOLUTION

A number of researchers have investigated the impact of temperature on local anaesthetic solutions. Interest has largely focused on the following three characteristics:

1. Injection pain
2. Onset time of local anaesthetic block
3. Duration of local anaesthetic.

Warming the local anaesthetic solution has been shown to significantly reduce injection discomfort. This has led to the development of some novel devices to warm local anaesthetic cartridges although in truth the same can be achieved by placing ampoules in warm water. Conversely anaesthetic potency has been shown to be significantly increased at lower temperatures. The mechanism for this may be that lower temperatures are associated with reduced local blood flow thus reducing anaesthetic "wash out" from the nerve. Lower temperatures may also affect the binding of the anaesthetic molecule at the voltage-gated sodium channel.

The optimal temperature for a local anaesthetic has yet to be fully elucidated but somewhere between 37 and 42° C would seem to be appropriate (Chilvers 1993). The clinical value of increased potency with the injection of cooled local anaesthetic solutions at the expense of increasing injection pain are not to be encouraged.

INFECTION AND LOCAL ANAESTHETIC INJECTIONS

Common sense would suggest that injecting local anaesthetic into an infected area is not appropriate. There are two principal reasons for this. Firstly tissue pH is lowered in the presence of infection. Lower tissue pH favours dissociation of the anaesthetic solution towards the ionized form, which reduces the available free base. The free base is the lipophilic component, which is able to diffuse across the axon's lipid-soluble membrane.

Secondly there is the risk of spreading infection by direct injection. The needle becomes contaminated with bacteria from the initial injection and is then placed into nearby tissues risking contamination. The other mechanism of spread relates to the anaesthetic solution being deposited into an infected area and effectively spreading bacteria, which become diluted in it through the tissues.

For these reasons, where infection is present it is necessary to adopt a more proximal injection site well away from the infected area. This may even mandate a different anaesthetic technique altogether.

CROSS-INFECTION CONSIDERATIONS

Even minor medical interventions, such as local anaesthetic injections, can be associated with the risk of infection. Clinicians should always assume potential contamination by facultative pathogenic, but potentially highly virulent, germs, although the patient may appear asymptomatic. Although some authors had produced evidence that questions the value of preinjection skin antisepsis it is the authors' contention that this represents current best practice and must form part of every anaesthetic injection protocol. Any rapidly acting antiseptic agent is appropriate for this purpose.

In addition to preinjection skin antisepsis consideration must be given to the protection of the anaesthetist and any assistants. Whilst gloves offer little by way of protection from the needle, most patients bleed after injections thus justifying the use of nonsterile gloves at all times. Furthermore we know that bacterial contamination of gloves is less than that of the ungloved hand.

Implementing use of only disposable equipment, in this context syringes in place of reuseable dental-type syringes, reduces risk by eliminating the disassembly of equipment after use in addition to the potential risks of failures in the sterilization processes.

SKIN TENSION

At all times when the needle enters skin it does so with greater efficiency and less trauma to the patient if the skin around the injection site is held taut. Allowing the skin to become loose as the needle approaches the skin is guaranteed to increase your patient's misery.

ANGLE OF NEEDLE ENTRY

In contrast to the technique of cannulation, where the approach angle of the needle is low, when injecting local anaesthetic solutions, the needle should be introduced at right angles to the skin. This will greatly reduce the initial pain of injection and make needle penetration easier. Figure 7.1 shows the correct angle for needle entry and Fig. 7.2 the incorrect angle.

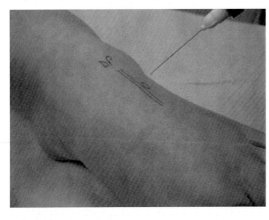

FIGURE 7.1
Correct needle entry into the skin.

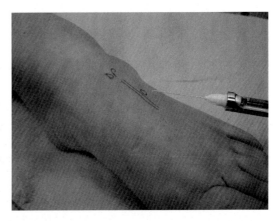

FIGURE 7.2
Incorrect needle entry into the skin.

PATIENT POSITIONING

This is largely determined by the type of block being administered. Do give due consideration to your patient's comfort especially when commencing blocks, which may take some time to complete.

For reference, various positions are described in Figures 7.3 to 7.6.

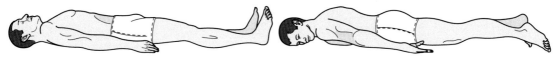

FIGURE 7.3
Supine position.

FIGURE 7.4
Prone position.

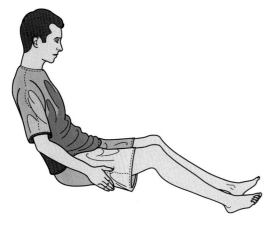

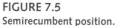

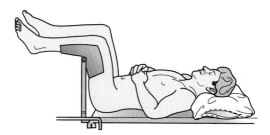

FIGURE 7.5
Semirecumbent position.

FIGURE 7.6
Lithotomy position.

REFERENCE

Chilvers, C.R., 1993. Warm local anaesthetic – effect on latency of onset of axillary brachial plexus block. Anaesth. Intensive Care 21, 795–798.

BIBLIOGRAPHY AND FURTHER READING

Albert, C., Brocq, O., Gerard, D., et al., 2006. Septic knee arthritis after intra-articular hyaluronate injection. Two case reports. Joint Bone Spine 73, 205–207.

Bader, L., et al., 2005. Bacterial infections following injections and infusion caused by errors of hygiene – how to avoid them. MMW Fortschr. Med. 147, 28–29, 31–32.

Dabarakis, N., et al., 2006. The role of temperature in the action of mepivacaine. Anesth. Prog. 53, 91–94.

Lieffers, M.A., Mokkink, H.G., 2002. Disinfection of the skin prior to injections does not influence the incidence of infections; a literature study. Ned. Tijdschr. Geneeskd. 146, 765–767.

Nallamshetty, L., Buchowski, J.M., Levon, A., et al., 2003. Septic arthritis of the hip following cortisone injection. Case report and review of the literature. J. Clin. Imag. 27, 225–228.

Yang, C.H., et al., 2006. Warm and neutral tumescent anesthetic solutions are essential factors for a less painful injection. Dermatol. Surg. 32, 1119–1122; discussion 1123.

BASIC LOCAL ANAESTHETIC TECHNIQUES

8

LOCAL INFILTRATION

See Table 8.1 for local infiltration.

Table 8.1 Local infiltration

Indications	Local infiltration of local anaesthetic is widely used in dermatological practice for the removal of superficial skin lesions. It is a simple technique to learn and highly effective for the treatment of lesions limited to the skin and subcutaneous tissue
Contraindications	Local infection Ischaemia Lesions to the plantar of the foot
Anatomy	Irrespective of anatomical location this block is effective because the surgical site is surrounded by a field of local anaesthetic solution thereby blocking the cutaneous nerves within this area
Anaesthesia	The area of anaesthesia will be determined by the location of the infiltration
Equipment	1 pair nonsterile gloves Skin wipe 1 × 10 mL disposable syringe 1 × 27 gauge needle
Drug	Any of the amide local anaesthetic drugs may be selected.
Volume	Between 5 and 10 mL of anaesthetic solution is usually required dependent upon the size of the skin area to be anaesthetized
Special considerations	Do not inject in to infected areas as there is a risk of spreading infection through the tissues Do not inject directly into skin lesions Avoid injury to local veins as this can cause substantial bruising
Vasoconstrictors	The application of a vasoconstrictor will greatly enhance the local haemostasis and is almost always advised with infiltration technique

TECHNIQUE: DORSUM OF THE FOOT

See Table 8.2 and Fig. 8.1 for dorsum of the foot.

Table 8.2 Dorsum of the foot

Position	The patient should be sat comfortably in a semirecumbent position with the leg straight
	FIGURE 8.1 Technique: dorsum of the foot.	The lesion marked in blue can be anaesthetized by beginning the injection at point A. A line of anaesthetic solution is deposited as the needle is directed towards point B Now the needle is withdrawn almost completely and then redirected towards point C whilst again depositing a small volume of anaesthetic solution as the needle advances • The final stage is to remove the needle and place a line of anaesthetic solution between points C–B

TECHNIQUE: POSTERIOR OF HEEL

See Table 8.3 and Fig. 8.2 for posterior of heel.

Table 8.3 Technique: posterior of heel

Position	The patient should be prone for infiltrations to the heel or posterior of the leg
	FIGURE 8.2 Technique: posterior of heel.	• The lesion illustrated here is innervated by the sural nerve. The options for anaesthesia would be either a local infiltration or a sural nerve block. The infiltration is readily performed by injecting anaesthetic solution from point A to B and then from A to D. A further two injections from point C to B and then C to D ensure that the lesion will be completely numb before treatment is instigated. Were the lesion positioned more plantarly then infiltration would be less desirable as the injection sites would be approaching the plantar skin. Direct injection into thick plantar skin is painful and should be avoided whenever possible

DIGITAL BLOCK

See Table 8.4 for digital block.

Table 8.4 Digital block

Indications	The digital block is a technically easy block to master and requires little specific training though good technique will minimize the trauma to the patient and enhance reliability. The block is indicated whenever it is necessary to achieve anaesthesia of a single digit distal to the metatarsophalangeal joints. Typical indications would be: • Cauterisation of warts/verrucae • Nail surgery • Subungual exostectomy
Contradications	• Local infection • Digital ischaemia
Anatomy	Sensation to the hallux is provided by four main digital nerves: two dorsal and two plantar. Both plantar nerves are derived from the medial plantar nerves and provide innervation to the dorsal toe tip
Anaesthesia	The entire digit is rendered anaesthetic following successful digital block
Equipment	• 1 pair nonsterile gloves • Skin wipe • 1 × 5 mL disposable syringe • 1 × 27 gauge needle
Drug	Any of the amide local anaesthetic drugs may be selected with little variation in onset times as even with the slow-acting anaesthetic drugs such as bupivacaine and ropivacaine, onset is rapid. Anaesthesia should be achieved within a matter of 2–5 min as the digital nerves are small and well confined, thus diffusion distance of local anaesthetic solution is low
Volume	In most instances 3–5 mL of local anaesthetic solution is sufficient to achieve anaesthesia
Special considerations	Post injection skin necrosis has been observed where excessive volumes of anaesthetic solution were used resulting in pressure necrosis. It is important to avoid placing a complete ring of anaesthetic solution around the toe as this can potentially cause vascular compromise
Vasoconstrictors	Current guidance discourages the use of local anaesthetics with ephinephrine for digital anaesthesia in both hands and feet. Thompson et al. (2007) critically reviewed the evidence on which this current and persisting dogma is based. It appears that most of the cases in which digital ischaemia developed following administration of local anaesthetic and epinephrine occurred pre 1950 and utilized procaine or cocaine as the primary anaesthetic agent (both of which are vasoconstrictors). Sylaidis and Logan prospectively assessed the impact of digital anaesthesia using 2% lignocaine with 1:80000 epinephrine digital blocks on various parameters of digital arterial blood flow in 100 consecutive patients. Their findings demonstrated that epinephrine only temporarily reduced digital blood flow. Perfusion of the digits persisted in every case. A word of caution to the reader – whilst there is evidence that local anaesthetics with epinephrine in digital anaesthesia are not necessarily correlated with impending digital ischaemia, evidence from studies on the hand is not directly applicable to the feet, which are at the end of the circulatory line

HALLUX DIGITAL BLOCK TECHNIQUE

See Table 8.5 for hallux digital block technique.

Table 8.5 Hallux digital block technique

Position	The patient should be sat comfortably in a semirecumbent position with the leg straight
Step 1	The toe to be anaesthetized is held firmly either side. Fingers must not be located under the toe so as to minimize the risk of needlestick injury. Skin tension is achieved by bending the toe downwards into slight plantar flexion
Step 2	The needle enters at the dorsolateral side of the hallux. A small volume of anaesthetic solution is deposited within the subcutaneous tissue (Fig. 8.3)
Step 3	The needle is advanced towards the plantar surface of the digit taking care not to go all the way through the toe. Whilst advancing the needle, deposit a small volume of solution. With the operator's thumb away from the tip of the needle and the needle just in the subcutaneous tissue plantarly, deposit a further small volume of anaesthetic being sure to observe the skin under the toe blanche (Fig. 8.4)
Step 4	The needle is now withdrawn almost completely and then reorientated medially whilst remaining in the subcutaneous tissues (Fig. 8.5)
Step 5	The needle is now advanced towards the dorsal medial digital nerve and a small trail of anaesthetic solution is deposited as the needle is advanced. Once completed the needle is removed ready for the second injection point Note that using this technique the patient has only endured one injection point so far. As the skin at the second injection point is now numb the second injection should be pain free
Step 6	The final step is similar to the first injection. A small trail of anaesthetic solution is deposited as the needle advances plantarly. Once again, aim to observe skin blanching with the final anaesthetic deposit at the plantar medial aspect of the hallux (Fig. 8.6)

HALLUX BLOCK SEQUENCE (FIGS 8.3–8.6)

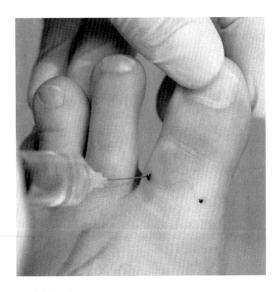

FIGURE 8.3
Hallux block sequence step 2.

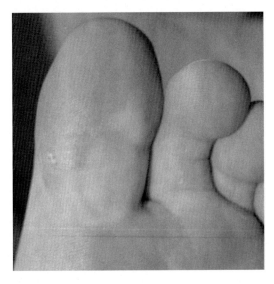

FIGURE 8.4
Hallux block sequence step 3.

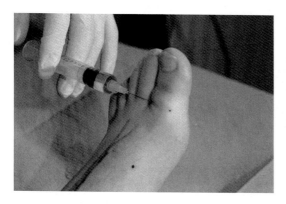

FIGURE 8.5
Hallux block sequence step 4.

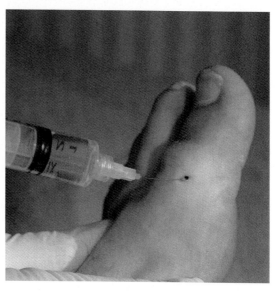

FIGURE 8.6
Hallux block sequence step 6.

INAPPROPRIATE TECHNIQUES

See Table 8.6, Figs 8.7, and 8.8 for inappropriate techniques.

Table 8.6 Inappropriate techniques

FIGURE 8.7 Inappropriate technique. 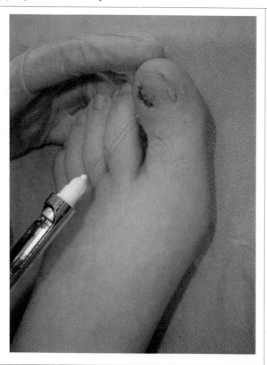	Injecting directly into the infected area is poor practice. It is painful, risks spreading infection, and due to local pH is less likely to work. The correct approach is to inject away from the infected area and perform a proper digital block rather than attempting infiltration

Continued

Table 8.6 Inappropriate techniques—cont'd

FIGURE 8.8 Inappropriate technique.	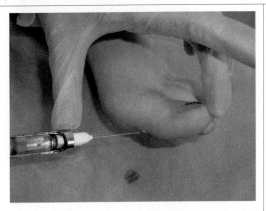	Injecting through the base of the digit is painful and unnecessary. The correct approach for the plantar digital nerves is from the dorsum

MAYO BLOCK

See Table 8.7 for Mayo block.

Table 8.7 Mayo block

Indications	The "Mayo block" is a type of field block used to anaesthetize a defined segment of the foot. It has no real advantages over the more refined technique of ankle block anaesthetic. The Mayo block is typically reserved for intraoperative "rescue" anaesthesia where access to more proximal nerve block is problematic usually as a result of surgical draping restricting access. The technique involves multiple injections to effectively block the sensation to a segment of the foot
Contraindications	• Local infection • Ischaemia
Anatomy	The local anatomy will vary according to the anatomical location. As the Mayo block is typically reserved for the first and fifth rays one can think of the innervation arising from each corner of an imaginary quadrant at the level of the block
Anesthesia	The area of anaesthesia will be determined by the location of the Mayo block administered. In general there are three segments: medial 1st ray, central rays, and 5th ray
Equipment	• 1 pair nonsterile gloves • Skin wipe • 1–2 × 10 mL disposable syringe • 1 × 27 gauge needle
Drug	Any of the amide local anaesthetic drugs may be selected. It is more beneficial to utilize a higher volume and lower concentration for the Mayo field block so as to maximize spread of anaesthetic solution
Volume	Between 10 and 15 mL of anaesthetic solution is usually required
Special considerations	This field block can be painful for the patient in comparison to other techniques. The effectiveness and duration of anaesthesia are also less in comparison to other techniques and it is therefore advisable to limit the application of this technique for "rescue anaesthesia" intraoperatively
Vasoconstrictors	There are no contraindications to the use of local anaesthetic drugs with vasoconstrictors

TECHNIQUE: MAYO BLOCK 1st RAY SEGMENT

See Table 8.8 and Fig. 8.9 for Mayo block 1st ray segment.

Table 8.8 Technique: Mayo block 1st ray segment

Position	The patient should be sat comfortably in a semirecumbent position with the leg straight.
	FIGURE 8.9 Technique: Mayo block 1st ray segment.
Step 1	Begin the injection at point A introducing local anaesthetic solution as the needle is passed plantarly to point B. Approximately 3 mL of anaesthetic solution is required for this component part of the Mayo field block. Note that the injection remains in the subcutaneous tissue at all times
Step 2	Withdraw the needle almost completely before redirecting to point C on the dorsal surface. This injection is also purely subcutaneous. A similar amount of anaesthetic solution is required
Step 3	The needle is now withdrawn completely and reinserted at position C, nearly but not quite at the base of the first metatarsal. If you begin the second injection too proximally it will not be possible to pass the needle to the plantar surface of the foot between the 1st and 2nd metatarsal. This injection will block the deep peroneal nerve dorsally and the plantar nerve at its deepest point. As the needle is directed plantarly a further line of anaesthetic solution is administered taking care to aspirate each time
Step 4	Because innervation to the medial segment will enter the field from the lateral side it is useful to place a line of anaesthetic solution from dorsal proximal (C) to dorsal distal (E). This is again a subcutaneous injection that will block any branches of the superficial fibular nerve
Step 5	The final injection passes from the plantar proximal portion of the 1st ray (B) across the sole of the foot to point D on the plantar lateral aspect of the 1st ray. This injection aims to block the plantar nerves supplying the 1st ray segment

ANKLE BLOCK

INDICATIONS

The technique is useful in any situation where complete anaesthesia of the foot below the level of the malleoli is required. It will provide complete anaesthesia distal to the injection level including, joints, bone, subcutaneous tissue, and skin. A complete ankle block involving all peripheral nerves providing innervation to the foot is frequently not required. The ankle block anaesthetic may be subcategorized into:

1. Full ankle block
2. Medial ankle block (omission of the sural nerve block).

Innervation to the foot is by means of five peripheral nerves only one of which arises from the femoral nerve, the remaining four being the terminal branches of the sciatic nerve. Two of these nerves are deep (tibial and deep fibular nerves); the remainder lie superficially within the subcutaneous tissue. Where anaesthesia to the lateral border of the foot is not required the sural nerve component may be omitted.

Ankle Block
- Saphenous
- Posterior tibial
- Superior fibular
- Deep fibular
- Sural

We shall consider each individually so that the practitioner is then able to perform these blocks individually or in combination, depending on particular clinical circumstances. In deciding which peripheral nerves to block always remember to take account of anatomical variation and overlap of cutaneous supply between these nerves (Fig. 8.10).

FIGURE 8.10
Cutaneous innervations of the foot.

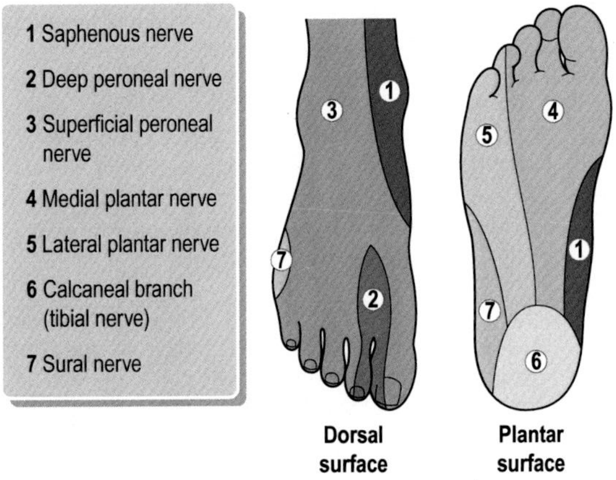

1 Saphenous nerve
2 Deep peroneal nerve
3 Superficial peroneal nerve
4 Medial plantar nerve
5 Lateral plantar nerve
6 Calcaneal branch (tibial nerve)
7 Sural nerve

Dorsal surface

Plantar surface

SAPHENOUS NERVE (L3,4)

ANATOMICAL COURSE

The saphenous nerve is the most distal continuation of the femoral nerve and descends in the thigh with the femoral artery deep to sartorius. At the posterior medial of the knee, it becomes subcutaneous and descends the leg with the great saphenous vein. The saphenous nerve provides sensation to the medial surface of the leg and foot up to the level of the first metatarsophalangeal joint. At the ankle, the nerve is easy to locate being adjacent to the great saphenous vein on the dorsal surface of the ankle (Figs 8.11 and 8.12). The nerve is subcutaneous throughout its course in the leg and provides sensation to the medial border of the foot (Table 8.9).

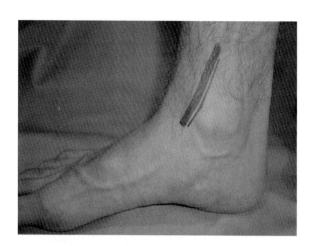

FIGURE 8.11
Anatomical location of the saphenous nerve.

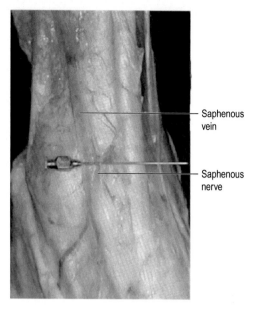

Saphenous vein

Saphenous nerve

FIGURE 8.12
Saphenous nerve.

Table 8.9 Saphenous nerve

AREA OF SKIN INNERVATION	MUSCLE SUPPLY
Medial border of the foot and medial arch up to the level of the 1st metatarsophalangeal joint	The saphenous nerve does not provide any muscle innervation

SAPHENOUS NERVE (ANKLE) – (L3,4)

See Fig. 8.13.

FIGURE 8.13
Saphenous nerve – cutaneous supply.

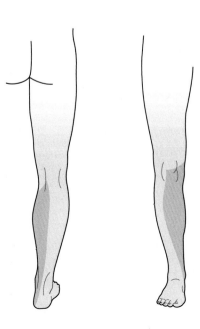

INJECTION TECHNIQUE

Although the nerve is easy to identify and should therefore be able to be blocked with a small volume of anaesthetic, in clinical practice the author prefers to begin the injections at the site of the nerve and continue it medially (Fig. 8.14). This ensures that any small branches will be blocked, thereby ensuring adequate anaesthesia. If there is difficulty in finding the saphenous vein one can apply a light tourniquet to the leg around the calf and place the limb dependent (hanging down). This allows for easy identification of the vein as it becomes filled with blood. The tourniquet must be applied lightly and removed immediately after identification.

FIGURE 8.14
Saphenous nerve – cutaneous supply injection technique.

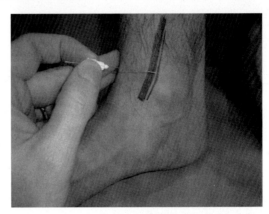

SAPHENOUS BLOCK

See Table 8.10 for saphenous block.

Table 8.10 Saphenous block

Indications	Blockade of the saphenous nerve at the level of the ankle is indicated for: • Surgical procedures involving the medial side of the foot • Diagnostic nerve block of the saphenous nerve
Contraindications	• Local infection • Active local venous ulceration
Anatomy	At the level of the ankle the saphenous nerve lies adjacent to the great saphenous vein within the subcutaneous tissue. The nerve is easily accessible at this site for PNB. Care should be take to avoid inadvertent intravascular injection
Anaesthesia	Blockade of the saphenous nerve at the ankle will afford anaesthesia of the skin along the medial aspect of the foot extending to the 1st metatarsophalangeal joint
Equipment	• 1 pair nonsterile gloves • Skin wipe • 1 × 5 mL disposable syringe • 1 × 27 gauge needle
Drug	Any long-acting amide local anaesthetic
Volume	In most instances 3–5 mL of local anaesthetic solution is sufficient to achieve anaesthesia
Special considerations	Avoid accidental intravenous injection due to the close proximity of the saphenous vein
Vasoconstrictors	When using a long-acting local anaesthetic there are no advantages

TECHNIQUE

See Table 8.11 and Fig. 8.15 for saphenous block technique.

Table 8.11 Saphenous block technique

Position	The patient should be sat comfortably in a semirecumbent position with the leg straight or in slight flexion at the knee	
Step 1	FIGURE 8.15 Saphenous block injection technique.	The key anatomical landmarks are: • Medial malleolus • Great saphenous vein
Step 2		The injection is directed just medial to the saphenous vein at the level of the ankle After negative aspiration inject 2–5 mL of local anaesthetic solutions

TIBIAL NERVE (ANKLE) (L4,5,S1-3)

The posterior tibial nerve is the largest distal continuation of the popliteal nerve and courses around the medial malleolus under the flexor retinacula. The nerve is quite large at this point before it divides into its terminal branches of the calcaneal, medial, and lateral plantar (Table 8.12). The posterior tibial nerve provides sensory innervation to the sole of the foot and innervates the plantar intrinsic muscles.

Table 8.12 Tibial nerve

AREA OF SKIN INNERVATION	MUSCLE SUPPLY
The tibial nerve (at the level) of the ankle further divides into three main branches: • Calcaneal • Medial plantar • Lateral plantar The main calcaneal branch provides sensation to the underside of the heel medially. The medial and lateral plantar nerves provide innervation to the remainder of the sole of the foot	Flexor hallucis brevis Flexor digitorum brevis Abductor hallucis Adductor hallucis Abductor digiti minimi quinti Flexor accessorius

NERVE LOCATION

There are three acceptable techniques for location of the posterior tibial nerve block at the ankle:

1. Palpation of the nerve
2. Pulse location
3. Low-powered nerve stimulator.

The technique of 'needle paraesthesia' is no longer considered acceptable due to the risk of peripheral nerve damage. This technique involves advancing the needle towards the nerve until the patient reports paraesthesia along the distribution of the target nerve.

Palpation of the nerve

This is a useful technique in those 'skinny' individuals where there is minimal fat to impair palpation of the nerve. Standing over the patient place your index and middle fingers just behind the medial malleolus. Gently roll your fingers towards the malleolus whereupon you should feel a firm cord-like structure pass under your fingers. Sometimes this causes a paraesthesia to the sole of the foot confirming you have the correct structure located. Using this technique you are able to mark an approximate point on the skin under which the nerve lies.

Pulse location

A similar approach but this time you simply mark the position of the posterior tibial pulse behind the medial malleolus. You may do this using either your fingers or where the pulse is difficult using a Doppler unit prior to marking with a pen. Both of these techniques provide you with an approximate location of the nerve prior to injection. Remember the nerve lies just posterior to the vascular supply. After you have marked the vessel site place your fingers directly over the mark and aim to just miss your fingers with the needle aiming posterior to the vessels. The nerve lies quite superficial though below the flexor retinaculum. Remember to direct the needle from medial to lateral as you look at the foot. Sometimes there is a tendency for clinicians to aim posterior towards the Achilles tendon.

Note that the injection is placed just posterior to the vessel with the needle placed at right angles to the skin aiming towards the fibular malleolus (Fig. 8.16).

Please refer to Table 8.13 for more details.

FIGURE 8.16
Correct entry point of needle for posterior tibial block in relation to the vessels.

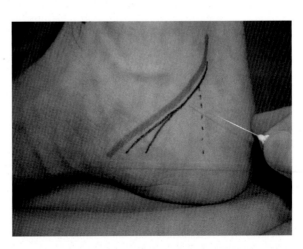

Table 8.13 Tibial nerve

Indications	The tibial nerve block is indicated in: • Isolated diagnostic nerve block • Surgical anaesthesia to the sole of the foot • Rescue analgesia
Contraindications	Local infection
Anatomy	The tibial nerve is located posterior to the medial malleolus just behind the vascular bundle. It lies deep to the flexor retinaculum
Anaesthesia	Anaesthesia may take 20 min to develop following injection. Failure to achieve anaesthesia of the heel is most often associated with placement error
Equipment	• 1 pair nonsterile gloves • Skin wipe • 1 × 5 mL disposable syringe • 1 × 27 gauge needle
Drug	Any of the amide local anaesthetic drugs may be used
Volume	In most instances 3–5 mL of local anaesthetic solution is sufficient to achieve anaesthesia
Special considerations	None
Vasoconstrictors	Will enhance the duration of anaesthesia when used in combination with the short- and medium-acting local anaesthetics

TECHNIQUE

See Table 8.14 for tibial nerve technique.

Table 8.14 Tibial nerve technique

Position	The patient should be sat comfortably in a semirecumbent position with the leg straight
Step 1	Manually locate the pulses with your index finger
Step 2	Introduce the needle just away from your finger tip posterior to the pulse and aiming towards the posterior of the medial malleolus
Step 3	After negative aspiration inject 4–6 mL of local anaesthetic solution slowly
Step 4	Allow 10–15 min before testing the block

SUPERFICIAL FIBULAR (PERONEAL) NERVE (L4,5; S1)

The superficial fibular nerve is one of two main terminal branches of the common fibular nerve arising at the level of the fibula neck. The nerve descends through the peroneal muscles providing innervations as it does so. The nerve becomes subcutaneous at the distal third of the leg before further branching into the intermediate and lateral dorsal cutaneous nerves (Figs 8.17, 8.18, and Table 8.15).

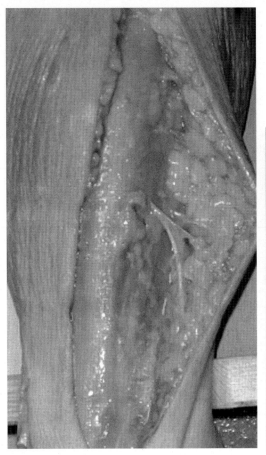

Lateral dorsal cutaneous nerve

Intermediate dorsal cutaneous nerve

FIGURE 8.17
Superficial fibular nerve.

FIGURE 8.18
Superficial fibular nerve at the ankle.

Table 8.15 Superficial fibular (peroneal) nerve (L4,5; S1)

AREA OF SKIN INNERVATION	MUSCLE SUPPLY
Dorsum of the foot except for the 1st toe cleft, which receives supply from the deep fibular nerve	This cutaneous nerve does not have any motor innervation

Whilst seemingly an attractive proposition, PNB at this juncture is impractical as it is difficult to locate the precise position at which the nerve pierces the deep fascia and becomes subcutaneous by clinical methods alone. The application of high-definition ultrasound would make such a technique possible.

Practically the two main branches of the superficial fibular nerve can be best located at the level of the ankle joint before they further divide into their terminal branches as they course distally. In some individuals these nerves can be visualized through the skin aided by plantar flexion of the digits. A good anatomical landmark is the tendon of tibialis anterior. The intermediate cutaneous nerve is approximately 1.5 cm lateral to this tendon.

SUPERFICIAL FIBULAR (PERONEAL) NERVE

See Table 8.16 for superficial fibular (peroneal) nerve.

Table 8.16 Superficial fibular (peroneal) nerve

Indications	The superficial peroneal nerve is appropriate for: • Isolated diagnostic nerve block • Surgical anaesthesia to the dorsum of the foot
Contraindications	Local infection
Anatomy	Becomes subcutaneous in the distal third of the leg where it subsequently divides above the ankle into: • Lateral dorsal cutaneous nerve • Intermediate dorsal cutaneous nerve
Anaesthesia	Anaesthesia is usually rapid in onset after injection as the nerves are small and subcutaneous. No more than 10 min should be required before testing this block
Equipment	• 1 pair nonsterile gloves • Skin wipe • 1 × 5 mL disposable syringe • 1 × 27 gauge needle
Drug	Any of the amide local anaesthetic drugs may be used
Volume	In most instances 5–7 mL of local anaesthetic solution is sufficient to achieve anaesthesia of both these nerves
Special considerations	None
Vasoconstrictors	Will enhance the duration of anaesthesia when used in combination with the short- and medium-acting local anaesthetics

SUPERFICIAL FIBULAR (PERONEAL) NERVE TECHNIQUE

See Table 8.17, Figs 8.19, and 8.20 for superficial fibular (peroneal) nerve technique.

Table 8.17 Superficial fibular (peroneal) nerve technique

Position	The patient should be sat comfortably in a semirecumbent position with the leg straight. The clinician is best positioned standing to the side of the limb to be anaesthetized
Step 1	**FIGURE 8.19** Superficial fibular (peroneal) nerve. The intermediate dorsal cutaneous nerve is roughly central to the point between the malleoli at the level of the ankle. The lateral dorsal cutaneous nerve lies approximately 1–2 cm in front of the lateral malleolus

Continued

Table 8.17 Superficial fibular (peroneal) nerve technique—cont'd

Step 2	FIGURE 8.20 Superficial fibular (peroneal) nerve technique.		Begin the injection centrally at the central point between the two branches. The needle should penetrate just into the subcutaneous tissue and no deeper
Step 3			A line of anaesthetic solution is then placed from medial to lateral thus capturing the main two branches and any further smaller nerve branches arising. As the anaesthetic solution is deposited it is usual to see the tissue swell from the deposition of anaesthetic solution. This will disperse within 10 min in most patients. Isolated block of either one of these nerves is possible if required. Plantar flexion of the foot and toes enhances visualization in some patients. The nerve is often felt as a hard cord-like structure, which can be palpated digitally

DEEP PERONEAL NERVE (L4,5 S1)

This nerve arises as one of two main branches of the common fibular nerve at the level of the neck of the fibular. It enters the anterior compartment of the leg via the anterior intermuscular septum to descend with the anterior tibial vessels over the interosseous membrane. The deep fibular nerve provides motor innervation to all of the muscles in the anterior compartment of the leg. At the level of the ankle joint the nerve lies between the tendons of extensor digitorum longus and extensor hallucis longus just medial to the dorsalis pedis artery. At this point the nerve further divides into two further smaller branches. The lateral branch passes to innervate the muscle of extensor digitorum brevis and further smaller branches provide innervation to the surrounding tarsal joints. The medial branch continues distally towards the first toe cleft before dividing into two terminal branches to supply cutaneous innervation to the 1st web space. The medial branch may also send a motor branch to the 1st dorsal interosseous muscle.

OVERVIEW OF MAIN BRANCHING OF THE DEEP FIBULAR NERVE (FIG. 8.21)

Along its course, the nerve provides innervation to the muscles in the anterior compartment of the leg. The nerve divides into its two terminal branches; it sends off articular branches to the ankle joint (Fig. 8.22).

The lateral terminal branch supplies the muscles extensor digitorum brevis and extensor hallucis brevis. Draves further describes three smaller branches arising from the lateral terminal branch (Fig. 8.23).

These branches are termed the second, third, and fourth interosseous nerves. According to Draves these small interosseous branches innervate some of the intertarsal and tarsometatarsal joints as well as supplying the second, third, and fourth metatarsophalangeal joints. The medial terminal branch runs distally, lateral to the dorsalis pedis artery, as a direct continuation of the deep peroneal nerve. In addition to providing sensory innervation of the web space, the nerve gives off articular branches to the first metatarsophalangeal joint. The nerve becomes superficial at the web space lying in the subcutaneous tissue. At the level of the metatarsophalangeal joints, the nerve divides in two to become the second and third dorsal digital proper nerves. The second dorsal digital nerve provides sensory innervation to the lateral side of the hallux whilst the third dorsal digital nerve provides sensory innervation to the medial side of the second toe.

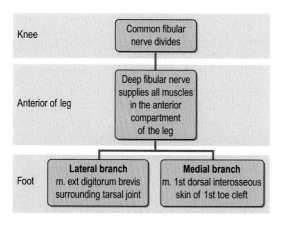

FIGURE 8.21
Overview of main branching of the deep fibular nerve.

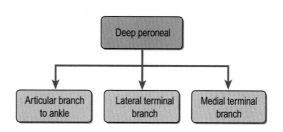

FIGURE 8.22
Division of the deep peroneal nerve.

FIGURE 8.23
Division of the lateral terminal branches of the deep peroneal nerve. MTP, metatarsophalangeal.

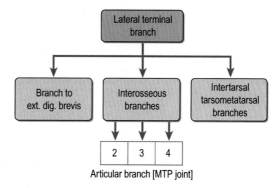

DEEP FIBULAR (PERONEAL) NERVE (FIG. 8.24)

See Table 8.18.

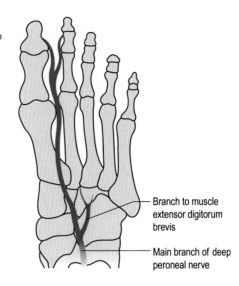

FIGURE 8.24
Anatomical location of the deep peroneal nerve.

Branch to muscle extensor digitorum brevis

Main branch of deep peroneal nerve

Table 8.18 Deep fibular nerve

AREA OF SKIN INNERVATION	MUSCLE SUPPLY
Distal to the ankle the deep fibular nerve provides sensory innervations to the first toe cleft and inside borders of the 1st and 2nd toes	Leg: • Extensor digitorum longus • Extensor hallucis longus • Tibialis anterior Foot – Provides innervations to two of the dorsal intrinsic muscles: • Extensor digitorum brevis • Extensor hallucis brevis • 1st dorsal interosseous

INJECTION TECHNIQUE (TABLE 8.19)

Table 8.19 Deep fibular nerve injection technique

Indications	The deep fibular nerve block may be indicated for: • Anaesthesia to the 1st web space • Diagnostic block • As a component part of the ankle block technique
Contraindications	Local infection
Anatomy	At the level of the ankle the nerve lies deep between the tendons of extensor hallucis longus and extensor digitorum longus. As the nerve travels distally it lies adjacent to the dorsalis pedis artery close to bone. Proximal injection at the level of the ankle or just below ensures the terminal branches are captured with the nerve block

Table 8.19 Deep fibular nerve injection technique—cont'd

Anaesthesia	Successful blockade provides anaesthesia of skin to the dorsum of the 1st toe cleft and is important in providing anaesthesia to the extensor digitorum brevis muscle and tarsal joints in this area
Equipment	• 1 pair nonsterile gloves • Skin wipe • 1 × 5 mL disposable syringe • 1 × 27 gauge needle
Drug	Any of the amide local anaesthetic drugs may be selected. Usually 5 mL of solution is adequate
Volume	In most instances 3–5 mL of local anaesthetic solution is sufficient to achieve anaesthesia
Special considerations	Care to avoid intravascular injection due to the close proximity of the local vasculature

Two levels of block are described for this nerve. They are the:

- Upper peroneal block
- Intermetatarsal block.

The upper peroneal technique being more proximal should provide anaesthesia to both the lateral and medial terminal branches. The more distal intermetatarsal block fails to block the lateral terminal branch, which arises proximal to the injection site. It is however usually adequate for surgeries around the distal metatarsal areas. The upper peroneal block is performed by locating the tendons of extensor hallucis longus and extensor digitorum longus. At the level of the ankle the deep peroneal nerve should lie approximately between these two structures. Insert the needle at right angles to the skin to a depth of approximately 1–2 cm; the needle should be aiming for the plantar surface of the foot and not the ankle joint. It is easy to misdirect the needle and end up depositing the anaesthetic into the ankle joint by mistake. If the needle is correctly positioned it will contact bone as it is advanced. After negative aspiration, deposit approximately 3 mL of anaesthetic. To improve the reliability of this block a fanning technique can be employed so that a greater spread of solution is achieved. This fanning technique simply involves withdrawal of the needle and redirection medially as it is once again advanced towards bone. When inserted to the desired depth, additional anaesthesia is deposited after negative aspiration. The procedure is then repeated, this time with the needle being directed laterally.

The distal technique (Fig. 8.25) is somewhat easier to perform and relies upon location of the dorsalis pedis artery, which lies medial to the nerve. Having located the artery, place the injection just lateral to it. The injection is placed deep to the subcutaneous tissues ensuring negative aspiration. As there may be some anatomical variation, it is useful to fan the injection from medial to lateral as described earlier, taking care to aspirate each time. It is essential to ensure the solution is deposited just above bone as the nerve lies deep to the deep fascia.

FIGURE 8.25
Distal block deep peroneal nerve.

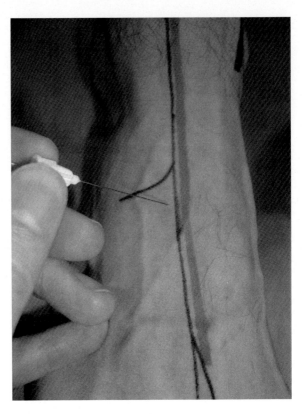

UPPER PERONEAL BLOCK TECHNIQUE

See Table 8.20 and Fig. 8.26 for upper peroneal block technique.

Table 8.20 Upper peroneal block technique

Position	The patient should be sat comfortably in a semirecumbent position with the leg straight	
Step 1		Locate the natural space between the tendons of extensor digitorum and hallucis longus just at the level of the ankle joint. This is aided by having the foot relaxed and in a dorsiflexed position. The space between these tendons is normally readily identifiable

Table 8.20 Upper peroneal block technique—cont'd

Step 2	FIGURE 8.26 Technique. Upper peroneal block.	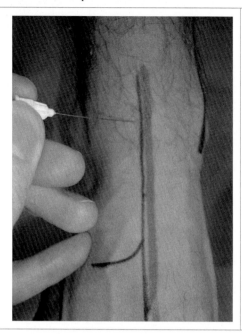	The needle entry is orientated towards the bone then withdrawn approximately 1 cm. After negative aspiration 5 mL of anaesthetic is administered in a fan-like direction to ensure adequate spread of anaesthetic solution

SURAL NERVE (S1,2) (FIGS 8.27, 8.28, AND 8.29)

The sural nerve arises from the tibial nerve within the popliteal fossa and communicating branch of the common fibularis muscle within the popliteal fossa. The nerve then descends on the posterior surface of gastrocnemius to enter the superficial fascia middle of the back of the leg. The sural nerve follows the course of the small saphenous vein supplying the lateral aspect of the lower leg and lateral border of the foot including the lateral border of the fifth toe.

See Tables 8.21 and 8.22 for sural nerve.

FIGURE 8.27
Origin of sural nerve.

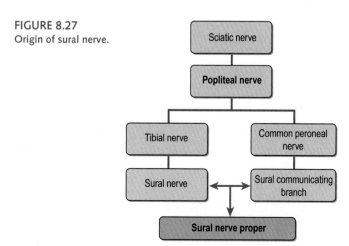

FIGURE 8.28
Sural nerve.

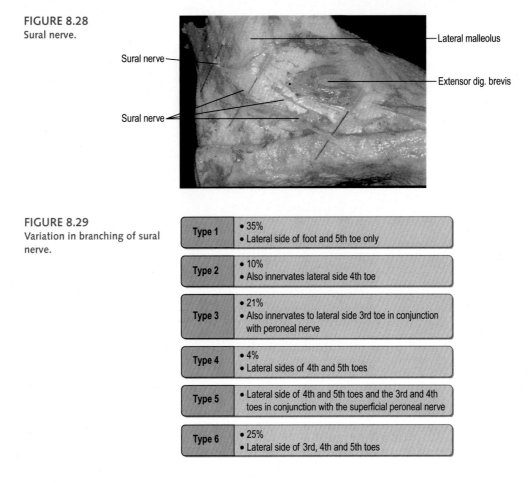

Sural nerve

Sural nerve

Lateral malleolus

Extensor dig. brevis

FIGURE 8.29
Variation in branching of sural nerve.

Type 1	• 35% • Lateral side of foot and 5th toe only
Type 2	• 10% • Also innervates lateral side 4th toe
Type 3	• 21% • Also innervates to lateral side 3rd toe in conjunction with peroneal nerve
Type 4	• 4% • Lateral sides of 4th and 5th toes
Type 5	• Lateral side of 4th and 5th toes and the 3rd and 4th toes in conjunction with the superficial peroneal nerve
Type 6	• 25% • Lateral side of 3rd, 4th and 5th toes

Table 8.21 Sural nerve (S1,2)

AREA OF SKIN INNERVATION	MUSCLE SUPPLY
The sural nerve arises within the popliteal fossa from cutaneous branches of both the tibial and common fibular nerves. It supplies the skin to the posterior lateral aspect of the lower one third of the leg and lateral border of the foot to the level of the 5th metatarsophalangeal joint	This cutaneous nerve does not have any motor innervation

Table 8.22 Sural nerve (S1,2)

Indications	This nerve block is indicated for: • Surgery to the dorsum (lateral to 3rd toe) and lateral border of the foot • Isolated diagnostic nerve block
Contraindications	Local infection
Anatomy	The nerve is subcutaneous and is readily located lateral to the Achilles tendon before it divides into multiple branches as it courses around the lateral malleolus

Table 8.22 Sural nerve (S1,2)—cont'd

Anaesthesia	Will afford anaesthesia to the lateral and dorsolateral border of the foot dependent upon the pattern of branching and overlap of innervation with the lateral dorsal cutaneous nerve. Also provides some innervation to the plantar lateral aspect of the heel
Equipment	1 pair nonsterile gloves Skin wipe 1 × 5 mL disposable syringe 1 × 27 gauge needle
Drug	Any of the amide local anaesthetic drugs may be selected
Volume	In most instances 5 mL of local anaesthetic solution is sufficient to achieve anaesthesia
Special considerations	Avoid injecting below the level of the lateral malleolus as this is more painful for the patient than in the more mobile skin just behind the lateral malleolus

SURAL NERVE TECHNIQUE

See Table 8.23 and Fig. 8.30 for sural nerve technique.

Table 8.23 Sural nerve technique

Position	The patient should be sat comfortably in a semirecumbent position with the leg straight. If the patient is particularly externally rotated injection can be aided by having the patient lay on their side	
Step 1	FIGURE 8.30 Sural nerve technique.	A line of local anaesthetic is placed from the lateral malleolus to the Achilles tendon. The injection is subcutaneous and requires only 3–5 mL of anaesthetic solution

BIBLIOGRAPHY AND FURTHER READING

Barbero, C., Gris, C., Puget, J., Samili, K., 2000. Ropivacaine infiltration for foot surgery. Ann. Francaises Anesth. Reanimation 19 (Suppl. 1), 84s, Abs R091.

Bollini, C.A., Cacheiro, F., 2006. Peripheral nerve stimulation. Tech. Reg. Anesth. Pain Manag. 10 (3), 79–88.

Clough, T.M., Sandher, D., Bale, R.S., Laurence, A.S., 2003. The use of local anaesthetic foot block in patients undergoing outpatient bony forefoot surgery: a prospective randomised controlled trial. J. Foot Ankle Surg. 42, 24–29.

Dhukaram, V., Kumar, C.S., 2004. Nerve blocks in the foot and ankle surgery. J. Foot Ankle Surg. 10, 1–3.

Doty, R., Sukhani, R., Kendall, M.C., et al., 2006. Evaluation of a proximal site and the use of nerve-stimulator-guided needle placement for posterior tibial nerve block. Anesth. Analg. 103, 1300–1305.

Draves, D.J., 1986. Anatomy of the Lower Extremity. Williams & Wilkins.

Enneking, F.K., 2005. Lower-extremity peripheral nerve blockade: essentials of our current understanding. Reg. Anaesth. Pain Med. 30, 4–35.

Friedman, H.E., Jules, K.T., Springer, K., Jennings, M., 1997. Buffered lidocaine decreases the pain of digital anesthesia in the foot. J. Am. Podiatr. Med. Assoc. 87, 219–223.

Hadžić, A., 2007. Textbook of Regional Anesthesia and Acute Pain Management, first ed. McGraw-Hill.

Jankovic, D., 2004. Regional Nerve Blocks and Infiltration Therapy. A Textbook and Colour Atlas, third ed. Blackwell, Berlin.

Kaloian G. Ouzounov., 2005. New nail block technique. J. Am. Podiatr. Med. Assoc. 95, 589–592.

Klein, S.M., Evans, H., Nielson, K.C., et al., 2005. Peripheral nerve block technique for ambulatory surgery. Anesth. Analg. 101, 1663–1676.

Kullenberg, B., Topalis, C., Resch, S., 2006. Ankle nerve block – perioperative pain relief in surgery of the forefoot. The Foot 16, 135–137.

Lennon, R.L., Horlocker, T.T., 2006. Mayo Clinic Analgesic Pathway. Mayo Scientific Press.

Marti, M.G., Muret, A.G., Nasif, L., et al., 2006. Ankle block for hallux valgus surgery: a comparison between 1.5% mepivacaine, 0.75% ropivacaine and 0.75% ropivacaine with nerve stimulation. Reg. Anaesth. Pain Med. 31 (5 Suppl. 2), 21, Abs 156.

Migues, A., Slullitel, G., Vescovo, A., et al., 2005. Peripheral foot blockade versus popliteal fossa nerve block: a prospective randomized trial in 51 patients. J. Foot Ankle Surg. 44, 354–357.

Radovic, P.M., Smith, R.G., Shumway, D., 2003. Revisiting epinephrine in foot surgery. J. Am. Podiatr. Med. Assoc. 93 157–160.

Rees, S., Tagoe, M., 2002. The efficacy and tolerance of local anaesthesia without sedation for foot surgery. The Foot 12, 188–192.

Rudkin, G.E., Micallef, T.A., 2004. Impediments to the use of ankle block in Australia. Anaesth. Intensive Care 32, 368–371.

Sarrafian, S.K., Ibrahim, I.N., Breihan, J.H., 1983. Ankle-foot peripheral nerve blocks for mid and forefoot surgery. Foot Ankle 4, 86–90.

Smith, D.W., Peterson, M.R., DeBerard, S.C., 1999. Local anesthesia. Topical application, local infiltration, and field block. Postgrad. Med. 106, 57–60, 64–66.

ADVANCED LOCAL ANAESTHETIC TECHNIQUES

9

SAPHENOUS NERVE BLOCK (KNEE)

See Table 9.1 and Fig. 9.1 for saphenous nerve block.

Table 9.1 Saphenous nerve block

Indications	The saphenous nerve is accessible for PNB either through blockade of the femoral nerve or in isolation just below the knee where it is subcutaneous. This PNB will provide anaesthesia to the medial, anterio-medial and posterior-medial aspect of the leg. Practically however, the large number of branches of the nerve at this point can make complete blockade challenging. If the sole purpose of the block is to provide surgical anaesthesia to the medial side of the foot then this is more easily achieved distally at the level of the medial malleolus • Surgical procedures to the leg normally when used in combination with other PNBs • Supplementation of incomplete femoral block • Varicose vein procedures
Contraindications	Local infection Digital ischaemia
Anatomy	FIGURE 9.1 Saphenous nerve block (knee). Infrapatellar branch The nerve becomes cutaneous at the knee after piercing the fascia between the tendons of gracilis and sartorius. The nerve then sends an infrapatellar branch to the knee before descending subcutaneously alongside the great saphenous vein. The anatomical landmarks for this nerve block are the tibial tuberosity and medial border of the medial head of gastrocnemius

Continued

Table 9.1 Saphenous nerve block—cont'd

Anaesthesia	See Fig. 8.14 The entire medial, antero-medial, and posterior-medial portions of the leg. The medial border of the foot extending to the 1st metatarsophalangeal joint. Some of the smaller saphenous nerve branches are easily missed and so patchy anaesthesia can be a potential problem with the high saphenous block
Equipment	• 1 pair nonsterile gloves • Skin wipe • 1 × 5 mL disposable syringe • 1 × 27 gauge needle
Drug	Any long-acting amide local anaesthetic
Volume	In most instances 5–10 mL of local anaesthetic solution is sufficient to achieve anaesthesia. Successful block requires a good spread of local anaesthetic solution and therefore it is better to select a lower concentration drug in favour of an increased volume
Special considerations	Compared with some of the other PNBs this injection is often reported by patients as being quite uncomfortable, more so than the popliteal block. This is because the needle is being directed through a large area of well-innervated subcutaneous tissue. A careful and considerate technique is recommended The most common complication with this block is incomplete anaesthesia. Owing to the proximity of the nerve to the great saphenous vein, care should be taken to avoid the vein and its branches, especially in those patients with varicosities. Accidental injection into the vein risks not only problems of toxicity but more commonly, substantial bruising
Vasoconstrictors	When using a long-acting local anaesthetic there are no advantages

TECHNIQUE

See Table 9.2 and Fig. 9.2 for saphenous nerve block technique.

Table 9.2 Saphenous nerve block technique

Position	The patient should be sat comfortably in a semirecumbent position with the leg straight or in slight flexion at the knee.	
Step 1	Prepare the skin with suitable antiseptic and note reference landmarks.	The key anatomical landmarks are: • Tibial tuberosity • Superior medial border of gastrocnemius
Step 2	**FIGURE 9.2** Saphenous nerve block (knee) technique. 	The injection begins just medial to the tibial tuberosity A line of anaesthetic is placed from this directed medially and slightly inferiorly towards the medial head of gastrocnemius

COMMON FIBULAR NERVE BLOCK (L4,5; S1,2) (TABLE 9.3)

The common fibular nerve (previously referred to as the common peroneal nerve) is the smaller of the two main branches of the popliteal nerve. It runs directly over the medial side of the tendon of biceps femoris and then winds around the neck of the fibular. As it curves around the fibular neck the nerve divides into the superficial and deep fibular (peroneal) nerves. The common fibular nerve is easily accessible for PNB at this point but this also renders it prone to injury.

Table 9.3 Common fibular nerve block (L4,5; S1,2)

Indications	Surgical anaesthesia to the leg in combination with other PNB Treatment of acute muscle spasm	
Contraindications	Local infection Digital ischaemia	
Anatomy	**Area of skin innervation**	**Muscle supply**
	Superficial fibular nerve provides sensory innervations to the distal one third of the leg anteriorly and the dorsum of the foot excluding the 1st toe cleft which receives it's sensory supply from the deep fibular nerve	Superficial fibular nerve innervates Muscles of lateral compartment of leg fibularis longus fibularis brevis
	The deep fibular nerve provides sensory innervation to the 1st toe cleft	Deep fibular nerve Muscles of anterior compartment of leg tibialis anterior extensor hallucis longus extensor digitorum longus fibularis tertius extensor digitorum brevis extensor hallucis brevis
Anaesthesia	Anaesthesia of the anterior and lateral aspect of the leg and foot in the muscles in the anterior and lateral compartment of the leg	
Equipment	• 1 pair nonsterile gloves • Skin wipe • Nerve stimulator • 1 × 5 mL disposable syringe • 1 × pole needle	
Drug	Any long-acting amide local anaesthetic	
Volume	In most instances 5 mL of local anaesthetic solution is sufficient to achieve anaesthesia	
Special considerations	The common fibular nerve is very superficial as it courses around the fibular neck and is easily traumatized during the PNB. There is a very real risk of serious nerve injury with this block. As such, careful patient counselling is advised and the block should only be performed by someone experienced in the technique	
Vasoconstrictors	When using a long-acting local anaesthetic there are no advantages	

TECHNIQUE

See Table 9.4 and Fig. 9.3 for common fibular nerve block technique.

Table 9.4 Common fibular nerve block technique

Position	The patient should be sat comfortably in a semirecumbent position with the leg in slight flexion at the knee
Step 1	**FIGURE 9.3** Common fibular nerve block (L4,5; S1,2) technique. Patella Head of fibula
Step 2	Standard aseptic precaution is required. Having carefully palpated the fibula head and marked its outline the nerve can usually be palpated just posteriorly. The needle should enter slightly away from the anticipated location of the nerve itself. Advance the needle towards the nerve with an initial current output of no more than 2 mA. Once motor activity is noted reduce the output and locate the optimum needle position in the usual manner

POPLITEAL NERVE BLOCK

The popliteal block is the technique of PNB at the level of the popliteal fossa, the diamond-shaped space behind the knee. The boundaries of the fossa are superiorly, medially by the semimembranosis and semitendinosis and laterally by the biceps femoris. Inferiorly the fossa is formed by the heads of gastrocnemius. The sciatic nerve divides into the tibial and common peroneal (fibular) branches near the apex of the popliteal fossa. In 75% of patients this bifurcation occurs within 10 cm of the popliteal crease (in 95% within 13 cm); in a few patients the nerves remain separate for their entire course throughout the thigh. The nerve itself is well separated from the popliteal artery and vein and lies lateral and superficial to these vessels. This accounts for the low risk of vascular puncture with this PNB when an appropriate technique is employed.

The advantage of the popliteal block is the ability to achieve profound anaesthesia of the entire lower leg (when combined with high saphenous block) which will afford maximal duration of anaesthesia/analgesia beyond that of spinal and more distal PNBs. The other major advantage is that unlike with spinal and sciatic block there is no loss of hamstring function, which would otherwise prevent post-operative mobilization. Patients thus enjoy a prolonged block that requires only one injection point and are still able to mobilize with knee stability maintained to a satisfactory level for same day discharge. The risk of vascular puncture is low with this technique as the nerve is superficial and lateral to the vein and artery.

INDICATIONS

- Surgery to the lower leg/ankle/foot
- Provision of prolonged post-operative analgesia
- Provision of muscle relaxation to leg/foot.

CAUTIONS/CONTRAINDICATIONS (TABLE 9.5)

- Local infection
- International normalized ratio (INR) >3.

Table 9.5 Popliteal nerve block cautions/contraindications

Infection	Infection following PNB is extremely rare. Nonetheless appropriate skin disinfection prior to injection coupled with aseptic precautions is recommended
Toxicity	Although relatively high volumes of local anaesthetic solution are used, the popliteal fossa is an area of mainly adipose tissue (of low vascularity). Absorption of local anaesthetic is therefore low. Care should however be observed during the injection to ensure negative aspiration and incremental injection
Haematoma	With careful technique this should not develop as the major vessels are distant from the target nerve. When using the lateral approach however injection through or into the hamstring muscle may result in haematoma formation
Vascular puncture	Avoid medial redirection of the needle, because the popliteal artery and vein are positioned medially and deeper to the popliteal nerve
Nerve injury	With the use of a nerve stimulator and careful injection technique this complication should not arise. Do not inject if: - The patient complains of excessive pain during injection - High injection pressures are noted - When stimulation is obtained at <0.2 mA current (100 μs)
Injury	Patients must be instructed on the care of the insensate extremity and the risk of injury due to the lack of motor power with resultant "drop foot"

LOCAL ANATOMY

Figures 9.4 to 9.6 illustrate the key anatomical landmarks. The most important landmarks are the popliteal crease and lateral hamstring tendon of biceps femoris. For the majority of anaesthetic approaches these are the only two landmarks necessary. Both are readily identified by having the patient lie prone and flexing their knee slightly or if using the lateral approach with the patient supine, ask them to try to flex their knee against resistance. For details of skin innervation and muscle supply see Table 9.6.

FIGURE 9.4
Cross-section of the proximal popliteal fossa.

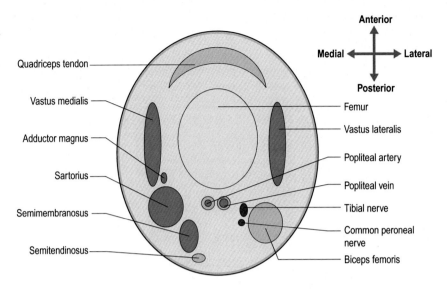

Quadriceps tendon

Vastus medialis

Adductor magnus

Sartorius

Semimembranosus

Semitendinosus

Anterior

Medial ← → Lateral

Posterior

Femur

Vastus lateralis

Popliteal artery

Popliteal vein

Tibial nerve

Common peroneal nerve

Biceps femoris

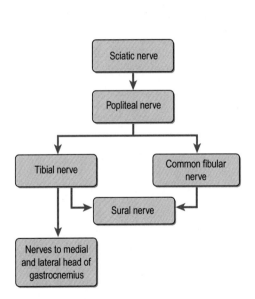

Sciatic nerve

Popliteal nerve

Tibial nerve

Common fibular nerve

Sural nerve

Nerves to medial and lateral head of gastrocnemius

FIGURE 9.5
Simplified branching of the popliteal nerve.

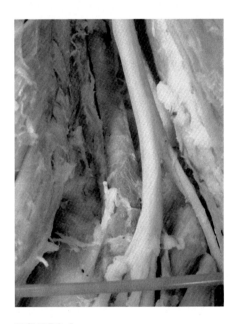

FIGURE 9.6
Rear dissection of right popliteal fossa showing popliteal nerve branching.

Table 9.6 Popliteal nerve

AREA OF SKIN INNERVATION	MUSCLE SUPPLY
Provides sensory innervation to the whole of the lower leg and foot through its branches with the exception of that supplied by the saphenous nerve	All muscles of the leg and foot through its various branches

EQUIPMENT

Irrespective of the approach chosen the equipment requirements are essentially similar (Table 9.7).

Table 9.7 Popliteal nerve block: equipment requirements

1	20 mL syringe 0.25% chirocaine
1	10 mL syringe 0.25% chirocaine
1	Nerve stimulator
1	Pole needle (50 mm)
1	ECG tabs
1	Skin prep
1	Nonsterile gloves
1	Assistant

ASEPTIC PRECAUTION

Although not strictly a sterile technique, measures to reduce the risk of cross-infection should be implemented including thorough skin disinfection prior to injection and the use of nonsterile gloves. Sterile draping is not necessary for this technique.

TECHNIQUES

There are three principal approaches to the popliteal block:

- Posterior approach
- Lithotomy
- Lateral.

The posterior approach is technically the easiest to teach and perform and has the advantage of a single needle entry point, which penetrates only skin and subcutaneous tissue as the needle is advanced toward the nerve. Because this approach requires the patient to be positioned prone it is not recommended for patients who are under general anaesthetic or heavily sedated unless the proposed procedure would require them to be positioned in this way.

The lithotomy approach is performed with the patient supine and the hip and knee flexed to 90°. This approach thus offers the advantage of not having to turn the patient. An assistant is required to stabilise the limb and in practice even slight movements can challenge even the most skilful operator. The needle entry is the same as for the posterior approach and is therefore easy to visualise with minimal risk of haematoma.

The lateral approach is performed with the patient supine and leg very slightly flexed. The approach is somewhat more painful for the conscious patient than the posterior or lithotomy approaches but it does have the advantage of being performed without the need to reposition the patient and avoids limb movement as is a problem with the lithotomy technique. Another drawback is the risk of haematoma that can occur with multiple needle passes.

POPLITEAL BLOCK: POSTERIOR APPROACH

Patient position

Position the patient prone with the leg fully exposed up to the thigh. Mark the leg to be anaesthetized and check carefully with the patient you have the correct limb. The foot must overhang the couch end so as to allow for dorsiflexion and plantar flexion of the foot during nerve stimulation. Cleanse the skin with an appropriate skin disinfectant.

Anatomical landmarks (Table 9.8, Figs 9.7, 9.8, and 9.9)

The most consistent landmarks are those of the tendons and popliteal crease. Attempts to visualize the imaginary diamond-shaped fossa as the basis of needle entry are fraught with error. Tendons are both consistent and easily palpable landmarks even in the weightier patient.

Table 9.8 Popliteal block technique

FIGURE 9.7 Popliteal block technique. 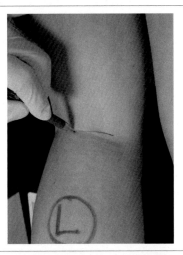	Begin by locating the popliteal crease and draw a line from medial to lateral **TIP:** This is aided by having the patient lift their foot, e.g., off the couch slightly
FIGURE 9.8 Popliteal block technique. 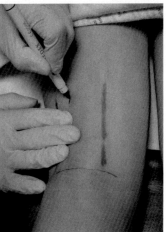	Next locate the medial and lateral hamstring tendons and mark their position carefully making sure you trace their course proximally at least 10 cm above the level of the popliteal fossa **TIP:** It is easier to begin marking these tendons from their insertion point then tracing proximally. Having the patient maintain their knee slightly flexed greatly assists with this

Table 9.8 Popliteal block technique—cont'd

FIGURE 9.9 Popliteal block technique. 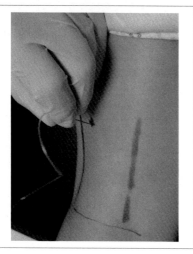	The needle is introduced approximately 7 cm (four finger breadths) above the level of the popliteal crease and 1 cm lateral to the midpoint between the tendons of biceps femoris laterally and semimembranosis and semitendinosis medially

Connecting the equipment

- Check the battery level of the nerve stimulator and ensure a spare is available
- Place ECG tab to either limb ensuring good surface to electrode contact. Remove hairs if present
- Connect the nerve stimulator to the skin electrode
- Connect the pole needle to the other lead using the clips as provided
- Finally attach the syringe containing local anaesthetic and run some fluid through
- If using a nerve stimulator with sensory and locate functions ensure the device is set to "locate" and that the leads are correctly connected.

Locating the nerve (Table 9.9)

The nerve stimulator should be set at about 2.5 mA output (or according to manufacturer's guidelines). Direct the pole needle vertically through the skin advancing slowly. Observe for contracture of the muscles supplied by either the tibial or common fibular branches of the popliteal nerve. Depending on the level of bifurcation stimulation of both branches may occur simultaneously.

When the desired muscle contracture is seen, reduce the output of the nerve stimulator and adjust the needle position until maximal muscle activity is seen with minimal mA output. Good muscle contraction with outputs of between 0.4 and 0.5 mA is an acceptable indication of adequate proximity to the nerve prior to injection.

Prior to injection check for negative aspiration. Checking intermittently for negative aspiration, inject the full 20 mL of local anaesthetic if stimulation of both nerve trunks is observed. If only one of the two branches is showing signs of stimulation inject only 10 mL of anaesthetic solution and proceed to step 5.

Table 9.9 Popliteal block: posterior approach

OBSERVATION	INTERPRETATION	ACTION
Simultaneous dorsiflexion, plantar flexion of foot and toes	Stimulation of both the tibial and common fibular components of the popliteal nerve	Optimal needle position subject to checking stimulation ceases below 0.2 mA as otherwise this might suggest intraneural needle position
Eversion and dorsiflexion of the foot with dorsiflexion of toes and plantar flexion of the 1st metatarsal	Stimulation of the common fibular nerve branch. Plantar flexion of the 1st metatarsal is due to contracture of peroneus longus and can be mistaken for stimulation of the tibial nerve	After blockade of the common fibular nerve it is recommended that the needle be redirected medially to locate the tibial branch of the popliteal nerve (double stimulation technique)
Plantar flexion of the foot at the ankle and flexion of the toes	Stimulation of the tibial nerve. It is essential to see both flexion of the foot and the toes as this ensures that the tibial nerve and not simply the motor branches to the gastrocnemius are being stimulated	After blockade of the tibial nerve it is recommended that the needle be redirected laterally to locate the common fibular branch of the popliteal nerve (double stimulation technique)
Plantar flexion of the foot at the ankle but no other movement	Most likely there is stimulation of the motor branches of the tibial nerve to the gastrocnemius muscle. This will not produce the desired sensory blockade	The needle position should be changed until activity of the long flexors and tibialis posterior is observed before proceeding with the injection
Contracture of the biceps muscle	This is most likely due to direct stimulation of the muscle itself. It can occur when the needle position is too lateral	Redirect the needle more medially until this muscle twitch ceases and direct stimulation of the main nerve trunk(s) is observed
Contracture of the semimembranosis muscle	This is most likely due to direct stimulation of the muscle itself. It can occur when the needle position is too medial	Redirect the needle more laterally until this muscle twitch ceases and direct stimulation of the main nerve trunk(s) is observed

Single versus double stimulation technique

In most cases stimulation of one or other of the two terminal branches will be observed. Some authors maintain that injection of a relatively large volume of local anaesthetic will lead to spread with the epineural sheath thereby providing anaesthesia to the other nerve branch. Others advocate location of the other nerve branch and subsequent blockade. This technique is more reliable and permits a reliable block with two injections of 10 mL of local anaesthetic.

Where initial stimulation of the tibial component is observed, the pole needle should be redirected laterally to locate the common fibular branch. This nerve may also be noted to be very slightly superficial to the tibial nerve. Once located correctly by observation of contracture of the peroneal muscles at an output of between 0.4 and 0.5 mA a bolus of 10 mL is administered in incremental steps after negative aspiration.

Needle advancement

It is useful to adopt a uniform strategy when attempting to locate nerves. The initial advancement should be in a vertical line from superficial to deep. Should you fail to locate the nerve withdraw the needle almost completely then angle medially before again advancing slowly. This may be repeated as required such that the needle covers a broad area.

Clinical tip – Do not be fooled by twitching of the hamstring muscles thinking this is the muscle activity you are seeking. Remember the muscle activity seen should be plantar flexion of the foot and toes for the tibial and dorsiflexion with eversion for the common fibular nerve. Contracture of the biceps muscle suggests the needle position is too lateral. Contracture of the medial hamstrings suggests the needle is too medial.

Auray 2002

Peripheral neuropathy seen in 1 of 952 blocks

Borgeat 2006

Series of 1001 continuous popliteal blocks:

- 0.5% paraesthesia nerve localization
- 0.8% pain on injection
- 0.4% blood on aspiration

Compere V 2005

Continuous popliteal/sciatic block for 5 days. Erythema noticed on removal. Subsequent deep absess. Meticillin-resistant *Staphylococcus aureus* (MRSA) identified

---

POPLITEAL BLOCK: LATERAL APPROACH

The lateral approach has the key advantage of allowing the patient to be left in a supine position and this is particularly important for those cases involving sedation or general anaesthesia. Consideration should also be given to this approach where patients have restricted mobility and may find moving into the prone position difficult. For those patients who are fully mobile and conscious for the performance of the block, the posterior approach is the preferred technique as it is less painful for the conscious patient.

Patient position

Position the patient supine with the knee flexed (30°–40°) as this aids location of the anatomical landmarks. The foot does not need to overhang the couch though it should be within easy view of the clinician injecting. The clinician should be seated on the same side and facing the limb to be injected. The limb should be marked in advance of the injection.

Tip – The limb should be maintained in a neutral position, i.e., patella facing directly upwards. Excessive internal or external rotation will alter the orientation of the nerve in relation to the needle direction.

Anatomical landmarks (Fig. 9.10)

As with the posterior approach it is best to rely upon osseous and tendon landmarks. In this instance the landmarks are:

- Patella
- Tendon of biceps femoris
- Iliotibial band
- Popliteal crease
- Vastus lateralis.

FIGURE 9.10
Popliteal block: anatomical landmarks for lateral approach.

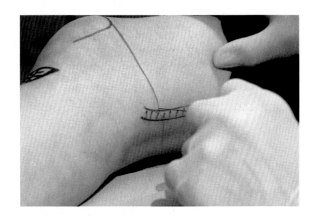

Connecting the equipment

As per standard.

Locating the nerve (Figs 9.11 and 9.12)

The entry point for this injection is determined by the intersection of the vertical line from the upper surface of the patella and the upper border of the tendon of biceps femoris. The needle thus passes through what is the muscle belly of the short head of biceps femoris. It should be angled horizontally.

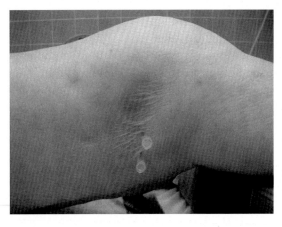

FIGURE 9.11
Popliteal block lateral approach: needle entry point.

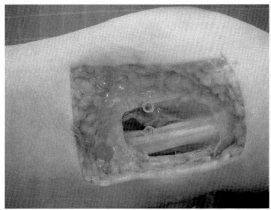

FIGURE 9.12
Popliteal block lateral approach: needle entry point.

Advance the needle through the bicep femoris into the popliteal fossa. As the needle advances contraction of this muscle should be seen. As the needle then advances, cessation of biceps muscle contraction indicates the needle tip is now within the popliteal fossa. When this point is reached the needle should be advanced slowly in anticipation of stimulation of the popliteal nerve. Stimulation of the common fibular nerve is noted first as this nerve lies lateral to the tibial branch. This is seen as dorsiflexion and eversion of the foot. Refinement of the needle position is carried out in the usual way to secure maximal motor response with minimal output (ideally 0.4–0.5 mA) When the optimal needle position is achieved a small test dose of anaesthetic is administered after a negative aspiration. Immediate cessation of motor activity further confirms correct positioning. The needle is then advanced further to locate the tibial nerve. The distance between the two nerves varies (5–25 mm). Approximately 10 mL 0.25% levobupivacaine has proven reliable with this technique.

Warning – Care should be taken to avoid excessive depth of needle penetration after cessation of the initial biceps muscle contraction is lost indicating entry of the needle tip into the popliteal fossa. Stimulation of the popliteal nerve is usually seen within a further 1–2 cm of needle advancement. Excessive needle advancement risks puncture of the popliteal vessels.

Danger zone of inappropriate needle placement

Placing the needle entry point too high, i.e., above the tendon of biceps femoris, will increase the risk of missing the nerve and potentially inadvertent vascular injury as the nerve is more superficial than the accompanying artery and vein. Thus as shown in Figures 9.13 and 9.14 the needle point 1 (Fig. 9.13) enters at almost the exact level of the nerve whereas the more anteriorly placed entry point 2 (Fig. 9.13) passes beneath the nerve and with sufficient advancement would directly impale the vessels.

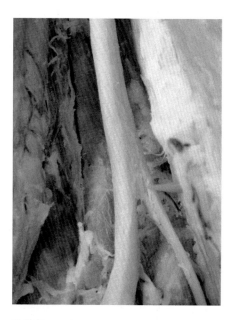

FIGURE 9.13
Danger zone of inappropriate needle placement.

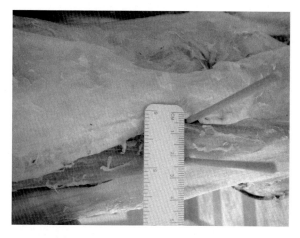

FIGURE 9.14
Danger zone of inappropriate needle placement.

POPLITEAL BLOCK: LITHOTOMY APPROACH

Patient position

Position the patient supine with the leg fully exposed up to the thigh. Mark the leg to be anaesthetized and check carefully with the patient that you have the correct limb. Cleanse the skin with an appropriate skin disinfectant. The limb needs to be held with the hip and knee flexed to 90°. An assistant supports the leg and thigh. The hip is held flexed at 90° and the knee should be flexed slightly to avoid excessive tension on the hamstrings whilst still allowing good visualization of the popliteal fossa. It is important the assistant maintains the limb in a steady position during the whole injection process.

Anatomical landmarks

The most consistent landmarks are those of the tendons and popliteal crease. Attempts to visualize the imaginary diamond-shaped fossa as the basis of needle entry are fraught with error. Tendons are both consistent and easily palpable landmarks even in the weightier patient. The landmarks are the same as for the posterior approach. Begin by drawing the popliteal crease, then the lateral hamstring tendon. Mark a point 7 cm proximal to the popliteal crease along the biceps tendon. The injection point is at this level 1 cm lateral to the midline of the leg.

Connecting the equipment

As per previous section.

Locating the nerve

It is essential that the assistant holds the limb completely still during the performance of this block. The nerve stimulator should be set at about 2.5 mA output (or according to the manufacturer's guidelines). Direct the pole needle vertically through the skin advancing slowly. Observe for contracture of the muscles supplied by either the tibial or common fibular branches of the popliteal nerve. Depending on the level of bifurcation stimulation of both branches may occur simultaneously.

When the desired muscle contracture is seen, reduce the output of the nerve stimulator and adjust the needle position until maximal muscle activity is seen with minimal mA output. Good muscle contraction with outputs of between 0.4 and 0.5 mA is an acceptable indication of adequate proximity to the nerve prior to injection.

Prior to injection check for negative aspiration. Inject a small amount (1–2 mL of local anaesthetic). Rapid cessation of the muscle contraction provides further indication of correct needle placement.

Checking intermittently for negative aspiration, inject the full 20 mL of local anaesthetic if stimulation of both nerve trunks is observed. If only one of the two branches is showing signs of stimulation inject only 10 mL of anaesthetic solution and proceed to step 5.

Single versus double stimulation technique

In most cases stimulation of one or other of the two terminal branches will be observed. Some authors maintain that injection of a relatively large volume of local anaesthetic will lead to spread with the epineural sheath thereby providing anaesthesia to the other nerve branch. Others advocate location of the other nerve branch and subsequent blockade. This technique is more reliable and permits a reliable block with two injections of 10 mL of local anaesthetic.

Where initial stimulation of the tibial component is observed, the pole needle should be redirected laterally to locate the common fibular branch. This nerve may also be noted to be very slightly superficial to the tibial nerve. Once located correctly by observation of contracture of the peroneal muscles at an output of between 0.4–0.5 mA, a bolus of 10 mL is administered in incremental steps after negative aspiration.

SPECIAL CONSIDERATIONS

Normal motor response to nerve stimulation may be diminished or even absent in a number of clinical circumstances. Attention should be paid to the presence of pre-existing conditions in the evaluation of response to nerve stimulation (Table 9.10).

Table 9.10 Popliteal block: special considerations

| Neuromuscular blocking agents | May be given as part of a general anaesthetic and will greatly diminish if not abolish any motor response dependent on the dose administered |
| Peripheral neuropathy | This rarely totally abolishes the motor response but the current required to evoke a motor response may be greater than usual. Where there is established neuropathy a target output current of 0.8–1 mA may be required to evoke a motor response |

SUCCESS RATES

The popliteal PNB is technically demanding: quoted success rates range from 80 to 99%. Interpretation of this variation is difficult since a number of authors utilize combined popliteal anaesthesia with some form of intravenous sedation/anxiolytic. Additional variation exists in the surgery to which these study groups are subjected. Clearly in such cases a less profound block in a patient under sedation may suffice whereas for the nonsedated patient it would not. In Author hands popliteal anaesthesia has a success rate of 95%. That is for every 100 cases done about 5 patients require additional anaesthesia or have to be rescheduled.

In the initial phases of developing this technique the overall success rate was more in the region of 80%. The introduction of popliteal anaesthesia to facilitate prolonged postoperative analgesia in patients not suitable for stronger opioids and/or NSAIDs increased Author's experience with this block with a resultant increase in success rate. In such patients in whom ankle block anaesthesia would suffice, the popliteal block was then administered initially. If there was inadequate anaesthesia with this, ankle block anaesthesia remained adequate to permit surgery to proceed. This is discussed then fully in the following section.

BIBLIOGRAPHY AND FURTHER READING

Badaoui, R, El Kettani, C, Yagoubi, A, et al., 2002. Combined sciatic-femoral nerve block: ropivacaine-clonidine mixture versus a bupivacaine-clonidine mixture. Eur. J. Anaesthesiol. 19 (Suppl. 24), 92, Abs A-355.

Bollini, C.A., Cacheiro, F., 2006. Peripheral nerve stimulation. Tech. Region Anesth. Pain Med. 10, 79–88.

Casati, A., Fanelli, G., Borghi, B., Torri, G., 1999. Ropivacaine or 2% mepivacaine for lower limb peripheral nerve blocks. Anesthesiology 90, 1047–1052.

Casati, A., Fanelli, G., Beccaria, P., et al., 2000. The effects of the single or multiple injection technique on the onset time of femoral nerve blocks with 0.75% ropivacaine. Anesth. Analg. 91, 181–184.

Casati, A., Fanelli, G., Magistris, L., et al., 2001. Minimum local anesthetic volume blocking the femoral nerve in 50% of cases: a double-blinded comparison between 0.5% ropivacaine and 0.5% bupivacaine. Anesth. Analg. 92, 205–208.

Casati, A., Borghi, B., Fanelli, G., et al., 2002. Double-blinded, randomized comparison of either 0.5% levobupivacaine or 0.5% ropivacaine for sciatic nerve block. Anesth. Analg. 94, 987–990.

Fernandez-Guisasola, J., Andueza, A., Burgos, E., et al., 2001. A comparison of 0.5% ropivacaine and 1% mepivacaine for sciatic nerve block in the popliteal fossa. Acta Anaesthesiol. Scand. 45, 967–970.

Jankovic, D., 2004. Regional Nerve Blocks and Infiltration Therapy. A Textbook and Colour Atlas, third ed. Blackwell, Berlin.

Klein, S.M., Evans, H., Nielson, K.C., et al., 2005. Peripheral nerve block technique for ambulatory surgery. Anesth. Analg. 101, 1663–1676.

Lennon, R.L., Horlocker, T.T., 2006. Mayo clinic analgesic pathway. Mayo Scientific Press, Rocherster, MN.

McLeod, D.H., Wong, D.H.W., Vaghadia, H., et al., 1995. Lateral popliteal sciatic nerve block compared with ankle block for analgesia following foot surgery. Can. J. Anaesth. 42, 765–769.

Marhofer, P., Oismuller, C., Faryniak, B., et al., 2000. Three-in-one blocks with ropivacaine: evaluation of sensory onset time and quality of sensory block. Anaesth. Analg. 90, 125–128.

Marti, M.G., Muret, A.G., Nasif, L., et al., 2006. Ankle block for hallux valgus surgery: a comparison between 1.5% mepivacaine, 0.75% ropivacaine and 0.75% ropivacaine with nerve stimulation. Reg. Anaesth. Pain Med. 31 (5 Suppl. 2), 21, Abs 156.

Peduto, V.A., Baroncini, S., Montanni, S., et al., 2003. A prospective, randomized, double-blind comparison of epidural levobupivacaine 0.5% with epidural ropivacaine 0.75% for lower limb procedures. Eur. J. Anaesthesiol. 20, 979–983.

Piangatelli, C., De-Angelis, C., Pecora, L., et al., 2004. Levobupivacaine versus ropivacaine in psoas compartment block and sciatic nerve block in orthopaedic surgery of the lower extremity. Minerva Anestesiol. 70, 801–807.

Provenzano, D.A., Viscusi, E.R., Adams, S.B., et al., 2002. Safety and efficacy of the popliteal fossa nerve block when utilised for foot and ankle surgery. Foot Ankle Int. 23, 394–399.

Santorsola, R., Casati, A., Carchierini, E., et al., 2002. A double-blind, randomised comparison of either 0.5% levobupivacaine, 0.5% ropivacaine or 0.5% bupivacaine for sciatic nerve block. Eur. J. Anaesthesiol. 19 (Suppl. 24), 94, Abs A-362.

Taboada, M., Cortes, J., Rodriguez, J., Ulloa, B., 2003. Lateral approach to the sciatic nerve in the popliteal fossa: a comparison between 1.5% mepivacaine and 0.75% ropivacaine. Reg. Anaesth. Pain Med. 28, 516–520.

Taboada, M., Alvarez, J., Cortes, J., et al., 2004. The effects of three different approaches on the onset time of sciatic nerve blocks with 0.75% ropivacaine. Anesth. Analg. 98, 242–247.

Urbanek, B., Duma, A., Kimberger, O., et al., 2003. Onset time, quality of blockade, and duration of three-in-one blocks with levobupivacaine and bupivacaine. Anaesth. Analg. 97, 888–892.

Vinciquerra, F., Casati, A., Borghi, B., et al., 2002. Levobupivacaine 0.5% or ropivacaine 0.5% for sciatic nerve block. Int. Monitor Reg. Anaesth. 14, Abs 25.

Vinciquerra, F., Speafico, E., Cappelleri, G., et al., 2003. Sciatic nerve block: a prospective, randomised, double-blind comparison between 0.75% ropivacaine and 0.75% levobupivacaine. Eur. J. Anaesthesiol. 20 (Suppl. 30), 109, Abs A418.

CORTICOSTEROID INJECTION THERAPY 10

INTRODUCTION

Silver (2007) reports that there are over eight million people in the UK suffering from some form of rheumatic disease and further estimates that approximately one fifth of all general practitioner consultations are for some form of rheumatological or musculoskeletal problem. Twenty percent of orthopaedic referrals are for foot and ankle problems and the use of corticosteroid injection therapy in the management of such problems is widely performed. As with the sections on local anaesthesia, this book is a practical guide; it is not meant to be a full and up-to-date distillation of the combined summation of the literature. A full critical review of the pros and cons in, for example, injection for Achilles tendonopathy, is therefore outside the scope of this book. However, key concepts and references are cited, and an extensive bibliography is supplied.

Accurate diagnosis using appropriate hospital and laboratory tests to confirm clinical findings is key to the appropriate and judicious use of injection therapy. It is worth reiterating that the practitioner must take a detailed and accurate history of the presenting illness (HPI) and have an excellent knowledge of anatomy before considering the use of corticosteroid therapy.

PHYSIOLOGY AND PHARMACOLOGY

Control of most body functions is achieved through the action of the nervous and endocrine systems, constituting the two main communication systems of the body. The endocrine system comprises primarily of the anterior and posterior lobes of the pituitary gland, the adrenal gland, the pancreas, the gonads (ovaries and testes), the thyroid, and the parathyroid glands. A hormone is a chemical secreted by a cell or group of cells into the blood for transport to a distant target, where it exerts its effect at very low concentrations. The term "steroids" refers to a group of naturally occurring hormones, synthesized mainly in the adrenal cortex and the gonads.

The adrenal glands are two small, triangular glands loosely attached to the kidneys (Fig. 10.1). They are divided into two morphologically distinct regions:

1. The adrenal cortex (outer)
   - zona glomerulosa (secretes aldosterone)
   - zona fasciculata (secretes glucocorticoids)
   - zona reticularis (secretes androgens)
2. The adrenal medulla (inner)
   - Secretes epinephrine and norepinephrine.

The two principal naturally occurring adrenal corticosteroids are:

- Aldosterone (a mineralocorticoid)
- Hydrocortisone/cortisol (a glucocorticoid).

Chemically, they are derived from cholesterol and the molecules share a common chemical structure. This similarity in the core structure of the compounds results in an

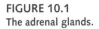

FIGURE 10.1
The adrenal glands.

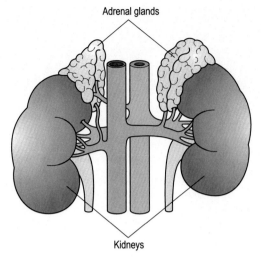

Adrenal glands

Kidneys

overlap of the activities of individual molecules. The name mineralocorticoid derives from early observations that these hormones were involved in the retention of the mineral sodium.

Adrenal corticosteroids have two distinct classes of action, referred to as glucocorticoid and mineralocorticoid activity:

1. Glucocorticoid activity affects carbohydrate and protein metabolism
2. Mineralocorticoid activity affects water and electrolyte balance.

Mineralocorticoids alter electrolyte and fluid balance by facilitating sodium reabsorption and hydrogen and potassium excretion at the level of the distal renal tubule, resulting in oedema and hypertension.

Glucocorticoids are characterized by an ability to bind with the glucocorticoid receptor. On reaching the target tissue, steroids cross the lipid membrane and bind to inactive glucocorticoid receptors, which exist in a complex with heat shock proteins in the cytoplasm. They exert their effects by modifying the rate of gene transcription and hence protein synthesis.

Physiologically, the glucocorticoids have a wide range of actions and glucocorticoid receptors are found in a wide range of tissues. As well as anti-inflammatory and immunosuppressive actions, they affect carbohydrate, protein and lipid metabolism, the cardiovascular system, and the central nervous system.

With overdosage or prolonged therapeutic use of corticosteroids, the normal physiological actions are exaggerated, causing side effects. For mineralocorticoids these include:

- Hypertension
- Sodium and water retention
- Potassium loss.

High doses of glucocorticoids can result in Cushing's syndrome.

Corticosteroids vary greatly in their ability to cross the placenta. Betamethasone and dexamethasone cross readily, however 88% of prednisolone is inactivated as it crosses. As a result of the reduction of the immunological response, patients using corticosteroids are at greater risk of infection and of severity of infection. Therefore, wherever possible, local treatment (creams, ointments, intra-articular injections, inhalations, eye-drops or enemas) should be used in preference to systemic treatment in order to reduce the likelihood of serious side effects. In inflammatory conditions of the joints, particularly in rheumatoid arthritis, they are given by intra-articular injection to relieve pain, increase mobility, and reduce pain and stiffness in one or a few joints (see Chapter 11). Full aseptic precautions are essential; infected areas should be avoided.

A list of common corticosteroids is given in Table 10.1 and see Figure 10.2 for a typical chemical structure (methylprednisolone).

Table 10.1 Common corticosteroids

GENERIC NAME	TRADE NAME	GLUCOCORTICOID POTENCY	MINERALO-CORTICOID POTENCY	DURATION OF ACTION ($t_{1/2}$ in hours)
Hydrocortisone	Hydrocortistab	1	1	8
Prednisolone	Deltastab	4	0.8	16–36
Methylprednisolone	Depo-Medrone*	5–7.5	0.5	18–40
Triamcinolone	Adcortyl (10 mg/mL) Kenalog (40 mg/mL)	5	0	12–36
Dexamethasone	Decradron	25–80	0	36–54
Betamethasone	Betnesol	25–30	0	36–54

*Available premixed with lidocaine hydrochloride 10 mg/mL.

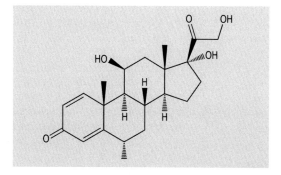

FIGURE 10.2
Methylprednisolone.
Reproduced from http://en.wikipedia.org/wiki/Image:Methylprednisolone.svg.

EVIDENCE FOR INJECTION THERAPY

Injection therapy is one of the most common therapeutic interventions in rheumatology. However, even though injectable steroids have been around for over 50 years, there is a paucity of good evidence regarding their use. The challenge is to apply the available evidence in a safe and effective manner. Injection therapy for the treatment of joint pain has been performed for many years using different substances. Compounds such as sodium bicarbonate, potassium phosphate, and procaine have been used from the first half of the twentieth century (Miller et al. 1958). Hollander et al. reported the use of hydrocortisone and cortisone in 1951 with further reports produced by Bornstein and Fallet, and Lambelet (cited by Miller et al. 1958). Since then, many studies have been produced discussing the use of steroid therapy for joint and soft tissue lesions but few studies meet the gold standard of a randomized controlled trial comparing the outcome of injection therapy with other treatments. Interpretation of the evidence is further compounded by a lack of consensus over diagnosis and outcomes measurement in the literature (Saunders & Longworth 2006).

Haslock et al. (1995) sent out questionnaires to 172 consultant rheumatologists to ascertain the techniques used for intra-articular and soft tissue injections. The results showed a wide divergence of practice in almost every aspect of the technique with respondents undertaking injections in almost any anatomical location. He concluded that there was a complete lack of consistency amongst British consultant rheumatologists. In a survey of general practitioners on joint and soft tissue injections, Liddell and colleagues found that nearly 65% of respondents had carried out injection therapy but that some had developed greater confidence and experience than others, with 51% of the injections being given by just 16% of practitioners (Liddell et al. 2005). Most general practitioners limited themselves to knee, shoulder and elbow injections.

Hayes et al. (2000) state that armed with a good knowledge of anatomy, proper injection technique and pharmacology, effective results are well within reach for the patient and clinician. Injectable corticosteroids deal with the problem at the site, delivering relief while eliminating adverse systemic effects with fewer potential complications than operative intervention.

As mentioned, a thorough review of the evidence for and against corticosteroid therapy is fascinating but outside the scope of this book. Practitioners are recommended to avail themselves of relevant literature to review and consider for and against the use of injectable steroids and more information is given in the sections on joint injections (Chapter 11) and soft tissue injections (Chapter 12). Saunders and Longworth have continued to amass the wealth of references as their injection therapy manual has been produced as a third edition (Saunders & Longworth 2006). Crawford and Thompson (2003) have looked at interventions for treating heel pain in their Cochrane Review of 2004 but practitioners should also review literature pertaining to knee, elbow, and shoulder pathology, which also contains a wealth of argument regarding the use of injection therapy (Assendelft 1996; van Der Heijden 1996). In recent years, podiatric surgeons, podiatrists, physiotherapists, and nurses have all gained access to the use of injection therapy (ACPOM 1999; Kriss 2003; Edwards et al. 2002), often under the use of a patient group directive. Given the relative safety, ease of use and cost-effectiveness of corticosteroid injection therapy, its use will continue to form a key part of the practitioner's armamentarium in modern clinical practice. One of the main barriers to achieving that competence is training and we hope that this text will add to the available knowledge base.

TREATMENT AIMS

The aim of treatment is to resolve pain and improve mobility and function. Individual professional bodies may set the requirements for their practitioners to perform such techniques, especially where the skill is acquired by postgraduate study.

The art of successful injection therapy is to place an appropriate amount of an appropriate drug into the correct location at the appropriate time. The practitioner must therefore consider:

- Diagnosis
- Anatomy
- Treatment algorithms
- Technique
- Drug choice
- Dosage.

DIAGNOSIS

Diagnosis is the process of identifying a medical condition or disease by its signs and symptoms, and from the results of various diagnostic procedures. An accurate diagnosis is the first step in the appropriate use of injection therapy. The use of diagnostic local anaesthesia has been emphasized at various points in this book.

ANATOMY

A sound knowledge of anatomy is key to injection therapy. This is crucial both for accurate diagnosis and proper needle placement. If a practitioner's knowledge of anatomy is poor they should not be seriously considering the use of injection therapy.

TECHNIQUE

The injection technique process is outlined later in this chapter.

TREATMENT ALGORITHMS

Injections can be a magic bullet for some patients but their use should be carefully considered as part of an overall treatment pathway or algorithm. For example, injection therapy certainly has a role in the treatment of plantar fasciitis but the injection of a dose of steroid should not be the first intervention offered to a patient that initially presents with heel pain. All too often, particularly in the UK, this is the case and may unfortunately be the first treatment offered by the generalist.

DRUG CHOICE

There are a range of drugs available to the practitioner but the broad considerations are with regard to soluble versus insoluble drugs and short-acting versus long-acting drugs. The author will give our recommendations in subsequent chapters.

DOSAGE CONSIDERATIONS IN PRACTICE

A typical rule of thumb will be to use small volumes of steroid for anatomically confined locations. For instance use a small volume of steroid for a small joint or use a larger volume of steroid in a larger joint. Also consider previous treatment; doses can be adjusted based on previous treatment. For example, if limited improvement has been given from a first dose of steroid, a higher dose might be considered for subsequent injections. Patient factors should also be considered including general hypersensitivity and occupational factors.

CONTRAINDICATIONS – SOFT TISSUE INJECTION RECOMMENDATIONS

- If the patient is pregnant or breast-feeding
- Overlying soft tissue infection, cellulitis or dermatitis
- A viral infection or TB
- Bacteraemia
- A known hypersensitivity to any of the constituent agents

- Lack of response after two injections
- Severe coagulopathy
- Anticoagulant therapy (relative contraindication).

CONTRAINDICATIONS – INTRA-ARTICULAR INJECTIONS

As for soft tissue, and:

- No more than three injections per year in weight-bearing joint
- Unstable joints
- Inaccessible joints
- Joint prosthesis
- Osteochondral fracture.

SIDE EFFECTS AND COMPLICATIONS

Systemic side effects include:

- Facial flushing: this may occur 24–48 hours after the injection, but will settle within a day or two
- Deterioration of diabetic glycaemic control
- Falls in inflammatory markers (ESR/CRP)
- Uterine bleeding
- Anaphylaxis.

Occasionally, but more commonly with the fluorinated compounds, an acute inflammatory reaction known as a steroid flare occurs. This happens in 10% of patients and may be a reaction to the microcrystalline suspension of the corticosteroid used, but must be distinguished from sepsis introduced into the injection site. Over-the-counter painkillers, such as paracetamol, can be taken if required by the patient. Fat wasting – a small amount of subcutaneous fat at the injection site – may be affected by the injection leaving an indentation at the injection site. Hypopigmentation may also be seen – this is of more concern to patients with a darker complexion. Soft tissue calcification, tendon rupture (see Chapter 12), joint sepsis, and steroid arthropathy have also been reported.

Poor outcomes with injection therapy arise with:

- Diagnosis
  - An inaccurate diagnosis is made
- Knowledge of anatomy
  - The drug is put into the wrong tissue
- Treatment algorithms
  - Steroid therapy is used inappropriately
  - Treatment is aimed at alleviating the symptoms without addressing the underlying cause
- Technique
  - Poor technique allows the spread of drugs into adjacent tissues
  - Injections are given too frequently
  - Little regard is given to aftercare
- Drug choice
  - An inappropriate drug is chosen
- Dosage
  - Too little or too large a dose is given.

TECHNIQUE AND PROCESS

INJECTION TECHNIQUE

1. Select the patient
2. Prepare the injection site
3. Prepare the injection
4. Give the injection
5. Record drugs/dosages/batch numbers
6. Give (and make a record of) aftercare advice.

SELECTING THE PATIENT

- Do you have a clear diagnosis?
- Is injection therapy the best treatment at this point in the treatment pathway?
- Discuss all the options
- Are there any contraindications (absolute or relative)?
- Warn about side-effects
- Record that this has been done.

Information to be given to the patient should include:

- The diagnosis and nature of their condition
- The details of proposed treatment and the alternatives
- The nature and effects of drugs to be given
- The most likely possible side-effects and incidence
- The likely benefits
- Your plans for follow-up and aftercare.

PREPARE THE INJECTION SITE

- Position the patient
- Mark the site
- Swab the skin and allow to dry (iodine is preferred for joint injections) – see also Chapter 5 on aseptic precautions
- Have cotton wool and plaster at hand.

All too often the clinician will swab the injection site and then re-contaminate the area by re-palpating the anatomy and/or joint margin. This is especially the case if the area was marked up prior to injection but the skin markings are erased with cleansing. A useful tip is to mark the injection site with a cross – the intersection of the cross is the injection point. If an alcoholic antiseptic is used, the centre of the cross will be erased but the injection point will still be visualized.

PREPARE THE INJECTION

- Decide the dose and volume
- Wash and dry hands
- Open vials/swab bungs
- Draw up the steroid
- Dilute with local anaesthetic: 50/50, depending on local guidelines and legislation
- Change the needle after drawing up solution(s).

RATIONALE FOR MIXING WITH LOCAL ANAESTHETIC

Saunders and Longworth (2006) suggest the following advantages of mixing steroid with local anaesthetic.

1. Diagnosis: this helps confirm the diagnosis and placement of the solution
2. Analgesia: although temporary, a reduction in pain will make the whole process less painful for the patient, may help break the pain cycle, and may reduce the post injection flare
3. Dilution: an increased volume of solution helps spread the active drug where a larger joint is being injected
4. Distension: large volumes of injected solution may help break down scar tissue and adhesions.

EQUIPMENT

- Syringes: use a 2.5 or 5 mL Luer lock syringe – the attachment of the needle to the syringe is much more secure
- Needles:
  - white (19 gauge)
  - green (21 gauge)
  - blue (23 gauge)
  - orange (25 gauge)
  - grey (27 gauge).

19 and 21 gauge needles are for aspiration and drawing up of fluid. The 23 gauge needle is the default setting to use for injecting but ensure that the needle length is adequate. The short 25 gauge needle is useful for superficial injections only. The 27 gauge needles can be too "whippy" such that the path of the needle is too easily deflected in trying to get the needle tip to the right spot.

CHOICE OF STEROID

The choice of which drug to use is guided by clinician preference for both drug and dose. We recommend:

- Soft tissue: use methyl prednisolone, hydrocortisone
- Joints: use triamcinolone

See Chapters 11 and 12 for recommended dosages.

GIVING THE INJECTION – STEPWISE APPROACH

1. Patient consent – can be oral or written, but must be *informed*
2. Use (nonsterile) gloves; gowns are not required
3. Keep talking to the patient – let them know what to expect
4. Apply strong skin traction using a nontouch technique
5. Insert the needle rapidly and perpendicularly to the skin
6. Attempt to aspirate
7. Inject joints and bursae as a bolus; entheses with a peppering technique
8. Withdraw needle gently and keep the plunger depressed to prevent suction of the steroid back into the syringe
9. Compress the site with cotton wool to prevent capillary leakage along the needle tract.
10. Dispose of sharps safely
11. Apply a dressing.

RECORD DRUGS/DOSAGES/BATCH NUMBERS

Record the technique and use of aseptic technique. Note and record:

- Name of drug used
- Dose
- Batch number
- Expiry date.

GIVE (AND MAKE A RECORD OF) AFTERCARE ADVICE

Inform and advice tell the patient that they should try to rest for the first 2–3 days after the injection and avoid any activities that normally make their symptoms worse. Side effects from the low doses used in injections are rare but can and do occur. Record what you told the patients in their notes. A patient information leaflet (PIL) can be useful but does not take the place of good oral communication.

EVALUATION OF INJECTIONS

Different practitioners follow different regimens following injections of steroids. The authors ask patients to rest for the first 2 days following injection, particularly when using insoluble corticosteroids such as triamcinolone as the first-line agent. These drugs tend to have more of an inflammatory response and the authors have found that when patients are less active following injections, this inflammatory flare is less aggressive. It may take days or weeks for the effects of the steroid to be noticed by the patient, especially if the patient experienced a flare. There is a wide range of views in the literature as to when to review the patient and if and when to re-inject. The authors schedule a review for 6 weeks post injection. When the patient returns there are a variety of scenarios that may have occurred:

1. The patient could be much improved. Patients may return reporting 90–100% improvement in symptoms. If performed in a joint, the steroid also works as a plasticiser and very often the patient will notice an increase in range of motion. At this point one can either discharge patients or keep them on a review-only basis.
2. If the patient is partially improved, one can consider a repeat infiltration. An element of experience is important as to how soon to perform the second injection, how much steroid to use, and whether to change the choice of drug. For those patients who are only moderately improved the authors will typically repeat the infiltration and review the patient in a further 6 weeks.
3. Where the patient shows no improvement, it is possible that the infiltration of steroid was not placed in the correct anatomical location. Consider use of image guidance (see Chapter 11).
4. Where the patient shows no improvement, it is possible that the diagnosis was wrong. For both these instances, review the patient history and consider the use of diagnostic nerve blocks.
5. Unfortunately, patients may return and have an increase in pain and symptomatology following an injection. This could be due to a severe steroid flare or it could be due to adverse trauma of the tissue from the tip of the needle. In these instances, even if the practitioner wants to re-inject, the patient may be disinclined to receive a further infiltration.

SUMMARY

In summary, the practitioner requires:

1. Accurate diagnosis
2. Sound judgement
3. Technical skills.

Without these, the results of injection therapy will be suboptimal. This means that the practitioner must reflect on whether they have developed competency in the use of injection therapy. Loeser (2004), in reviewing an article on saline injections in prolotherapy for back pain, writes:

Every needle has a sharp end that goes into the patient and a blunt end that is attached to a health care provider. Anyone who thinks that all the action occurs at the sharp end does not understand human behaviour.

REFERENCES

ACPOM, 1999. A Clinical Guideline for the Use of Injection Therapy by Physiotherapists. Chartered Society of Physiotherapists. Available at: http://www.csp.org.uk/director/members/libraryandpublications/csppublications.cfm?item_id=74C87795CDAE97F1ED4E232E019EF084.

Assendelft, W.J., Hay, E.M., Adhead, R., Bouter, L.M., 1996. Corticosteroid injections for lateral epicondylitis: a systematic overview. Br. J. Gen. Pract. 46, 209–216.

Crawford, F., Thomson, C., 2003. Interventions for treating plantar heel pain. Cochrane Database Syst. Rev. 3, CD000416.

Edwards, J., Hannah, B., Brailsford-Atkinson, K., et al., 2002. Intra-articular and soft tissue injections: assessment of the service provided by nurses. Ann. Rheum. Dis. 61, 656–657.

Haslock, Macfarlane, D., Speed, C., et al., 1995. Intra-articular and soft tissue injections: a survey of current practice. Rheumatology 34, 449–452.

Hayes Jr., D.W., Gilbertson, E.K., Mandracchia, V.J., Dolphin, T.F., 2000. Tendon pathology in the foot. The use of corticosteroid injection therapy. Clin. Pod. Med. Surg. 17 (4), 723–735.

Hollander, J.L., Brown Jr., E.M., Jessar R., Brown, C., 1951. Hydrocortisone and cortisone injected into arthritic joints; comparative effects of and use of hydrocortisone as a local antiarthritic agent. J. Am. Med. Assoc. 147, 1629–1635.

Kriss, S., 2003. Injectable steroids in the management of heel pain: a prospective, randomised trial. Br. J. Podiatry 6 (2), 40–42.

Liddell, W.G., Carmichael, C.R., McHugh, N.J., 2005. Joint and soft tissue injections: a survey of general practitioners. Rheumatology 44, 1043–1046.

Loeser, J.D., 2004. Point of view. Spine 29 (1), 16.

Miller, J.H., White, J., Norton, T.H., 1958. The value of intra-articular injections in osteoarthritis of the knee. J. Bone Joint Surg. 40B, 636–643.

Saunders, S., Longworth, S., 2006. Injection Techniques in Orthopaedics and Sports Medicine: A Practical Manual for Doctors and Physiotherapists, third ed. Elsevier, Edinburgh.

Silver, T., 2007. Joint and Soft Tissue Injection: Injecting with Confidence, fourth ed. Radcliffe Publishing, Oxon.

van Der Heijden, G.J.M.G., 1996. Corticosteroid injections for shoulder disorders: a systematic review of randomised clinical trials. Br. J. Gen. Pract. 46, 309–316.

BIBLIOGRAPHY AND FURTHER READING

Cole, B.J., Schumacher, H.R., 2005. Injectable corticosteroids in modern practice. J. Am. Acad. Orthop. Surg. 13, 37–46.

Derendorf, H., Möllmann, H., Grüner, A., Haack, D., Gyselby, G., 1986. Pharmacokinetics and pharmacodynamics of glucocorticoid suspensions after intra-articular administration. Clin. Pharmacol. Ther. 39, 313–317.

Haas, D.A., Carmichael, F.J.L., 2007. Principles of Medical Pharmacology, seventh ed. Elsevier, Canada.

Helliwell, P., Woodburn, J., Redmond, A., et al., 2007. The Foot And Ankle in Rheumatoid Arthritis. A comprehensive guide. Elsevier, Edinburgh.

Hussain, S., Durve, R., Brennan, S., et al., 2007. The chemical stability of admixtures of injectable corticosteroid and local anaesthetics. CME Orthopaedics 4, 81–83.

McNabb, J.W., 2005. A Practical Guide to Joint and Soft Tissue Injection and Aspiration. Lippincott, Williams and Wilkins, Philadelphia.

Patient Group Directions, 2004. A Practical Guide and Framework of Competencies for all Professionals Using Patient Group Directions. National Prescribing Centre. Available at: http://www.npc.co.uk/publications/pgd/pgd.pdf

Rang, H.P., Dale, M.M., Ritter, J.M., Flower, R.J., 2007. Pharmacology, sixth ed. Churchill Livingstone, China.

Rosenberg, J.N., Corticosteroid injections of joints and soft tissues. Available at http://www.emedicine.com/pmr/topic211.htm (updated Sept 2001).

Tallia, A.F., Cardone, D.A., 2003. Diagnostic and therapeutic injection of the ankle and foot. Am. Fam. Physician 68, 1356–1362.

COMMON FOOT AND ANKLE CONDITIONS: JOINT INJECTIONS

11

JOINTS

A joint is the junction between bones. Joints can be classified into three main categories:

1. Fibrous or fixed, e.g., the syndesmosis of the inferior tibiofibular joint
2. Cartilaginous, e.g., the pubic symphysis
3. Synovial, e.g., the first metatarsophalangeal joint.

OVERVIEW OF SYNOVIAL JOINTS

The bones of synovial joints are linked together by synovial capsules. Their ligaments may be intracapsular or extracapsular and the bones are covered by hyaline cartilage. A fibrous capsule usually encloses the joint completely. The capsule is lined throughout by a synovial membrane and the internal surfaces are lubricated by a viscous synovial fluid (Fig. 11.1).

FIGURE 11.1
The synovial joint.

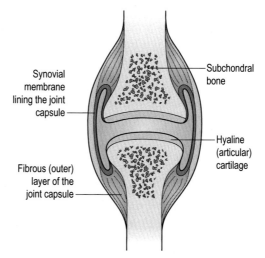

Synovial membrane lining the joint capsule

Subchondral bone

Hyaline (articular) cartilage

Fibrous (outer) layer of the joint capsule

ANATOMY

Articular surfaces are formed by specialized hyaline cartilage, which provides a wear-resistant, low-friction lubricated surface that is compressible and elastic and accommodates enormous forces of compression and shear during weight bearing and muscle action. The cartilage is closely moulded to bone, being thicker on central convex surfaces and thinning at the edges. Young cartilage is white and glistening, older cartilage becomes thinner and develops a yellowish appearance.

Synovial membrane lines the nonarticular parts of synovial joints. It is also found in synovial tendon sheaths and synovial bursae. The synovial membrane is smooth and moist and acts as a sieve: small molecules can pass through it to capillaries and venules and larger particulates pass into the lymphatics. The membrane does not coat any intra-articular discs or menisci. This membrane shows pathological changes in rheumatoid arthritis: it becomes thickened and secretes more fluid, resulting in swelling. The membrane contains elastin fibres, which impart a recoil in the membrane so that it does not become trapped in joint movement.

Synovial fluid is secreted by the synovial membrane and is found in the cavities of synovial joints, bursae, and tendon sheaths. Its viscosity, volume and colour vary between different joints and it shows viscous, elastic and plastic components, usually having an egg-like consistency ("synovial" partially derives from ovum, Latin for egg). Synovial fluid contains hyaluronan (hyaluronic acid), a polymer of disaccharides and lubricin (a water-soluble glycoprotein).

CLASSIFICATION OF SYNOVIAL JOINTS

1. Plain synovial joints, e.g., tarsometatarsal
2. Synovial hinge joints, e.g., interphalangeal
3. Synovial ellipsoid joint, e.g., metatarsophalangeal
4. Synovial ball and socket, e.g., hip, talonavicular
5. Synovial condyloid joints, e.g., knee
6. Synovial trochlear (saddle) joints, e.g., calcaneocuboid, ankle.

GENERAL CONSIDERATIONS

Intra-articular (IA) injections of corticosteroids are frequently used in the management of both osteoarthritis (OA) and rheumatoid arthritis (RA) despite the paucity of good-quality studies to assess their efficacy over placebo. Vanore et al. (2003) noted that judicious use of corticosteroid injections may provide rapid relief of pain even in recalcitrant cases, citing them as an initial treatment option for hallux rigidus. Tallia and Cardone (2003) stated that diagnostic aspiration or therapeutic injection of the ankle or first metatarsophalangeal joints can be performed for management of advanced osteoarthritis, rheumatoid arthritis, and other inflammatory arthritides such as gout or synovitis.

Ayral (2001), Gossec and Dougados (2006), and Ward et al. (2008) noted that most of the evidence for the efficacy of IA joint injection comes from the knee. Ayral and Gossec and Dougados suggest that the focus of IA should be short-term treatment of disease flares. Ward and colleagues (2008) conducted a prospective study to identify the long-term efficacy of corticosteroid injections in symptomatic foot and ankle joints and followed up patients at set intervals up to 1 year post injection. Using the Foot and Ankle Outcome Score questionnaire, they found statistically significant improved scores up to and including 6 months post injection with the magnitude of improvement at 2 months predicting the sustained improvement at 1 year. Solan et al. (2001) reported the results of manipulation under general anaesthesia (MUA) with injection of a depomedrone/bupivacaine mixture for hallux rigidus. In their cohort of 31 patients, patients with mild (grade 1) changes obtained relief for a median of 6 months with one third requiring surgery. Two thirds of patients with moderate disease (grade 2) proceeded to surgery and all patients with advanced hallux rigidus (grade 3) required surgery. The authors concluded that an MUA with corticosteroids should be performed for early and moderate disease. Although no patients were pain-free at 1 year, some stated that they would be happy to have further treatment.

It is common practice to mix the corticosteroid with a local anaesthetic prior to administration (Lavelle at al. 2007). The stability of methyl prednisolone when mixed with lidocaine has been assessed; however there is no evidence in the literature regarding the pharmacological stability of triamcinolone acetonide following admixture. Hussain et al. (2007) showed that the combinations of triamcinolone and hydrocortisone when mixed with combinations of lignocaine and bupivacaine are stable when mixed together as judged by high-performance liquid chromatographic (HPLC) analysis. Boxer (1994) states that when local anaesthetic is injected to anaesthetize the nerve supply to a joint it creates a chemical sympathetically resulting in dilation of the vessels feeding the synovia and capsule. The passive hyperaemia (inflammatory in nature) changes to an active hyperaemia and the inflammation is reduced. The reduction of pain removes the spasm and muscular guarding and the patient is more able to put the joint through the range of motion. This may help break down capsular adhesions and augment the anti-inflammatory effect of any steroid injected.

GUIDED INJECTIONS

Many authors acknowledge that without radiological confirmation, it is difficult to ensure the exact location of the needle, particularly in smaller joints. This is compounded by the potential for altered anatomy as seen with, for example, the reduced joint space and exostosis formation seen in OA. Khoury et al. (1996) found imaging studies to be less useful than diagnostic injections when attempting to identify the *source* of joint pain prior to arthrodesis. Adler and Sofka (2003) stated that injections based on anatomical landmarks can be accurate and that use of ultrasound to guide interventions in the musculoskeletal system, specifically the foot and ankle, will yield accurate placement of the needle tip for therapeutic injection and diagnostic aspiration. Fluoroscopic guidance is commonly used (Lucas et al. 1997; Newman 2003), especially by orthopaedic and podiatric surgeons. Saifuddin et al. (2005) felt that computed tomography (CT) provides a simple and safe alternative to fluoroscopy and may be the technique of choice for disordered anatomy. Author recommendation is to use some form of guidance for any joint injection proximal to the tarsometatarsal joint complex.

JOINT INJECTIONS

PAINFUL 1st METATARSOPHALANGEAL JOINT (TABLE 11.1 AND FIG. 11.2)

Table 11.1 Painful 1st metatarsophalangeal joint

Anatomy	The 1st metatarsophalangeal joint is a synovial joint comprised of four bones. The first metatarsal is the shortest and thickest of the five metatarsal bones. The distal surface or head of the metatarsal has a large cartilage-covered prominence, wider than the base of the proximal phalanx with which it articulates. On either side the cartilage overlaps onto the lateral aspect of the bone to form a smooth surface for the capsular ligaments of the joint. On the plantar surface of the head, there are two grooves for the articulation of the sesamoid bones, which are separated by the sesamoid ridge. The medial sesamoid and groove are larger than the lateral

Continued

Table 11.1 Painful 1st metatarsophalangeal joint—cont'd

Pathology	The most common clinical indication for a corticosteroid injection into the painful 1st metatarsophalangeal joint is mild to moderate osteoarthritis from hallux limitus (HL). HL can be defined as limitation of motion of the proximal phalanx at the first metatarsophalangeal joint in the sagittal plane to less than 65° dorsiflexion and less than 15° plantar flexion. The author has injected steroid into a 1st metatarsophalangeal joint for hallux abducto valgus on rare occasions only, and only then as part of an overall treatment plan to quell the worst of an inflammatory episode either prior to surgery or concurrently with orthotic therapy
	End-stage osteoarthritis is less amenable to the beneficial effects of steroid though its use can be considered – research and experience suggest that the results are better with mild and moderate disease. Ideally, the diagnosis is confirmed radiographically prior to injection. This is particularly helpful to identify the pattern of the disease and the potential presence of loose bodies thereby influencing the decision to inject
Equipment	2.5 or 5 mL syringe 25 mm (1 inch) 23 gauge (blue) needle
Drug(s)	20–40 mg of triamcinolone mixed with local anaesthetic
Positioning	The patient is typically positioned sitting up or supine, depending on patient preference
Technique (SEE VIDEO 12)	Map out the anatomical landmarks. The key structures to avoid are the long and short extensor tendons that are dorsally and dorsolaterally placed, respectively. The approach is through a dorsal medial incision, the needle entry point typically 0.5–1 cm medial to the extensor hallucis longus tendon. A medial approach is more painful and does not give as good access to the joint. The dorsolateral approach is deeper and more difficult overall. There is also a concern that leakage of steroid down the needle track from the dorsolateral approach will be close to the extensor hallucis brevis tendon
	Dorsiflex and plantar flex the toe and palpate the joint line. Distract the toe distally and look for puckering of the skin over the joint margins. Insert the needle perpendicularly to the skin and then change the angle to approximately 45° aiming distally and plantar laterally. Advance the needle, remembering the curvature of the joint. Aim to have at least half the length of the needle deep to the skin and be careful to do as little trauma to the cartilage of the base of the proximal phalanx as possible
Comments See PPS 12	Changes in joint morphology from cartilage erosion and osteophytosis can reduce the joint space and change the joint shape making the injection more difficult
	Patients normally experience positive results over the next few days but improvement may not be noticed for 2 weeks. The authors review patients after 6 weeks and will consider further injections as indicated

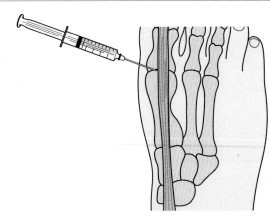

FIGURE 11.2
Painful 1st metatarsophalangeal joint. (After Saunders and Longworth, 2006, with permission.)

ARTHRITIS AND CAPSULITIS OF LESSER METATARSOPHALANGEAL JOINTS (TABLE 11.2 AND FIG. 11.3)

Table 11.2 Arthritis and capsulitis of lesser metatarsophalangeal joints

Anatomy	The lesser metatarsals are miniature long bones possessing a shaft, a base or proximal end, and a head or distal end. The lesser 4 shafts are often long and slender, slightly convex longitudinally on their dorsal surfaces and concave on their plantar surfaces. They are triangular in section and taper from base to head. The heads articulate with their own proximal phalanx by means of a convex articular surface, which extends further on the plantar surface than the dorsal surface. The sides of the head are flattened with a depression surmounted dorsally by a tubercule, which gives attachment to the collateral ligaments of the metatarsophalangeal joints. The plantar plate is the fibrocartilaginous structure that supports the ball of the foot, withstanding considerable compressive and tensile forces
Pathology	Lesser metatarsophalangeal joint osteoarthritis is quite common and is a common sequelae of trauma and osteochondrosis. However it also complicates many cases of metatarsalgia, hammer toe syndrome, and other forms of inflammatory arthritis. Inflammation of the lesser metatarsophalangeal joint is most commonly associated with long-standing hammer toe syndrome, particularly the second metatarsophalangeal joint that presents with chronic hyperextension of the proximal phalanx
Equipment	2.5 or 5 mL syringe 25 mm (1 inch) 23 gauge (blue) needle
Drug(s)	10–20 mg of triamcinolone mixed with local anaesthetic
Positioning	The patient is typically positioned sitting up or supine, depending on patient preference
Technique (SEE VIDEO 14)	Injection into the metatarsophalangeal joint can be very useful as part of the overall management of digital deformity. However, be wary of its use if subluxation or rupture of the joint is suspected Dorsiflex and plantar flex the toe and palpate the joint line. Distract the toe distally and look for puckering of the skin over the joint margins. Insert the needle from a dorsomedial approach (to avoid the EDB tendon) perpendicularly to the skin and then change the angle to approximately 45° aiming distally and plantar laterally. Advance the needle, remembering the curvature of the joint. Aim to have at least half the length of the needle deep to the skin and be careful to do as little trauma to the cartilage of the base of the proximal phalanx as possible
Comments	The lesser metatarsophalangeal joint is much smaller than the first metatarsophalangeal joint and the approach is more difficult. It is also much more difficult to be confident that the needle is in the joint especially if the metatarsophalangeal joint is retracted

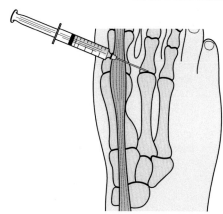

FIGURE 11.3
Arthritis and capsulitis of lesser metatarsophalangeal joints. (After Saunders and Longworth, 2006, with permission.)

TARSOMETATARSAL PAIN (LISFRANC'S JOINT) (TABLE 11.3 AND FIG. 11.4)

Table 11.3 Tarsometatarsal pain (Lisfranc's joint)

Anatomy	The tarsometatarsal joint is a complex of articulations between the metatarsals, the three cuneiforms, and the cuboid. The first 3 metatarsals articulate with the cuneiforms; the 4th and 5th metatarsals articulate with the cuboid. The 1st joint has an independent articular capsule and synovial cavity. The 2nd and 3rd joints have synovial cavities, which are continuous with the intermediate and lateral cuneiform, intercuneiform, cuneonavicular, and cuneocuboid joints. The 4th and 5th metatarsals have synovial cavities with the cuboid. An interosseous ligament crosses the base of the 4th metatarsal and the lateral cuneiform to shut off the cavities from one another. The bones are connected by dorsal and plantar tarsometatarsal and interosseous ligaments
Pathology	A common cause of pain is from osteoarthritis of the mid foot. Arthritis is more common in the first three metatarso-cuneiform joints and is typically associated with pronatory foot types and previous trauma. The typical mechanism of injury of a Lisfranc's joint is forced dorsiflexion, possibly from stepping off a kerb, but it is also associated with various sports, particularly horse riding (from the foot being caught in the stirrups). Fractures and fracture dislocations can be missed due to the difficulty in identifying subtle traumas and secondary OA can often follow missed primary trauma
Equipment	2.5 or 5 mL syringe 25 mm (1 inch) 23 gauge (blue) or 27 gauge (grey) needle
Drug(s)	10–20 mg of triamcinolone mixed with local anaesthetic
Positioning	The patient is typically positioned sitting up or supine, depending on patient preference
Technique	Where patients present with pain that is limited to the dorsum of the foot, they often respond well to steroid injection. It is normally fairly easy to identify an exostosis if present: mark it up and take a relatively vertical approach and aim to ensure that the needle is placed intra-articularly. A thinner gauge needle is often useful for this injection. A larger or irregular exostosis complicates the insertion of the needle into an already tight joint space and therefore the "whippiness" of the 27 gauge (grey) is a rare advantage. As an alternative, the joint can be approached from an acute angle of approach – almost parallel to the metatarsal – to have the needle slide under the capsule and sit just over the joint line to pepper steroid just under the capsule. If this fails – consider use of diagnostic imaging See Fig 11.4
Comments	What is more challenging is when patients present with more advanced whole joint arthritis. It can be difficult to be sure which joint or joints are affected and appropriate diagnostic imaging should be used in the diagnostic process. Owing to the often complex clinical picture, consider diagnostic infiltrations of local anaesthetic first. Where whole joint or joints need to be injected this is best performed under an image intensifier. Although it is possible to successfully perform intra-articular injections in clinic, the authors do not recommend this to the less experienced injector

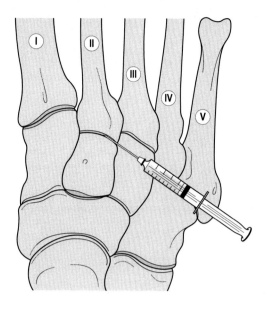

FIGURE 11.4
Tarsometatarsal pain (Lisfranc's joint). (After Saunders and Longworth, 2006, with permission.)

SINUS TARSI SYNDROME (TABLE 11.4 AND FIG. 11.5)

Table 11.4 Sinus tarsi syndrome

Anatomy	The calcaneus is the largest of the tarsal bones and projects posteriorly from the bones of the leg where its posterior surface gives insertion for the muscles of the calf. It is cuboidal in shape and its long axis points forwards, upwards, and slightly laterally. The anterior dorsal third is partly articular and partly nonarticular. The articular surface consists of middle and anterior facets for the talus, which extend forward and laterally and cover the dorsal surface of the sustentaculum tali. This surface may be divided into two by a narrow channel. Between the middle and posterior facets is a groove called the sulcus calcanei corresponding to the sulcus tali in the talus – together they form the sinus tarsi (tarsal sinus). This groove is directed in an anterolateral direction and opens out laterally into a rough quadrangle – the medial opening in the canalis tarsi. The anatomical space between the posterior and middle subtalar joint and is occupied by a talocalcaneal ligament, vasculature and nerves
Pathology	Pain and tenderness on the lateral side of the hind foot originating from the area of the sinus tarsus is known as sinus tarsi syndrome. It may follow injury of the talocalcaneal ligament after an inversion injury
Equipment	2.5 or 5 mL syringe 25 mm (1 inch) 23 gauge (blue) needle
Drug(s)	10–20 mg of triamcinolone mixed with local anaesthetic
Positioning	The patient is typically positioned sitting up or supine depending on patient preference, with the foot slightly supinated to open the sinus tarsi

Continued

Table 11.4 Sinus tarsi syndrome—cont'd

Technique	Injections of steroid into the sinus tarsi can be very useful. Consider use of a diagnostic local anaesthetic block first.
	Mark out the anatomy, particularly the peroneal tendons and the extensor digitorum brevis muscle belly. Feel for the dell of the sinus tarsi and insert the needle in a proximal-medial direction, following the direction of the sulcus.
	This is one of the few times when one needs to insert the needle to the end of the needle hub to ensure that one is as far in the sinus tarsi as possible. Obviously at this point the clinician needs to be concerned about the potential for needle breakage
	See Fig. 11.5
Comments	The large lateral opening of the sinus tarsi should be easy to locate but novice injectors are recommended to consider appropriate diagnostic imaging

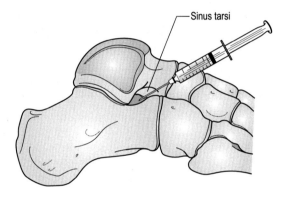

FIGURE 11.5
Sinus tarsi
syndrome. (After
McMinn, 2004, with
permission.)

— Sinus tarsi

REAR FOOT JOINTS (TABLE 11.5 AND FIG. 11.6)

Table 11.5 Rear foot joints

Anatomy	Anatomical subtalar joint: the talocalcaneal joint is a transverse cylindrical joint between the concave surface of the talus and the convex surface of the calcaneus. The posterior facets of the talus and the calcaneus are shut off from the other talocalcaneal facets by the interosseous ligament in the sinus tarsi
	The talocalcaneonavicular joint is a multi-axial ball and socket synovial joint. The convex head of the talus fits into the concave surface of the navicular. On the calcaneus, the talus articulates with the anterior and middle facets, which lie above the sustentaculum tali. The calcaneocuboid joint is a saddle-shaped synovial joint between the anterior surface of the calcaneus and the posterior surface of the cuboid. The cuboido-navicular joint is a fibrous joint
	Functional subtalar joint: all the facets of the subtalar aspect are involved. Therefore the posterior, middle and anterior facets of the talus and calcaneus make up the **functional** subtalar joint and have nothing to do with synovial cavities
	Functional midtarsal joint: the head of talus with navicular and head of calcaneus with cuboid make up the mid-tarsal joint in its functional aspect. Note that it is composed from 2 synovial cavities

Table 11.5 Rear foot joints—cont'd

Pathology	Arthritis of the talonavicular, calaneocuboid and subtalar joints is commonly seen, particularly following trauma, fracture, or end-stage inflammatory arthritis. Appropriate diagnostic imaging is key and therapeutic injections are best performed under image intensifier
Equipment	2.5 or 5 mL syringe 25 mm (1 inch) 23 gauge (blue) needle
Drug(s)	10–40 mg of triamcinolone mixed with local anaesthetic
Positioning	The patient is typically positioned sitting up or supine with the leg internally rotated, depending on patient preference and the joint to be injected
Technique	Mark out appropriate anatomy. Use of an image intensifier is necessary to ensure needle placement See Fig. 11.6
Comments	Not recommended for the novice injector

FIGURE 11.6
Rear foot joints.
(After McMinn,
2004, with
permission.)

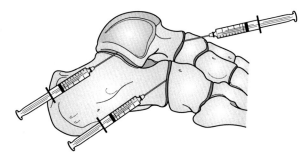

THE ANKLE JOINT (TABLE 11.6 AND FIG. 11.7)

Table 11.6 The ankle joint

Anatomy	The ankle joint is a hinge joint formed by the lower end of the tibia and its malleolus, the malleolus of the fibula, and the inferior transverse tibio-fibular ligament, which together form a deep recess into which the talus fits. The upper articular or trochlear surface of the talus is convex from front to back and concave from side to side. It is wider in front than behind. It is also curved slightly so that the concavity of the curve is directed medially. This medial angulation means that the front moves from slight abduction and dorsiflexion to a slight adduction and plantar flexion; wedging of the trochlear surface creates stability
Pathology	Primary ankle arthritis is rare but is seen secondary to trauma and previous fractures
Equipment	2.5 or 5 mL syringe 25 mm (1 inch) 23 gauge (blue) needle
Drug(s)	20–40 mg of triamcinolone mixed with local anaesthetic

Continued

Table 11.6 The ankle joint—cont'd

Positioning	The patient is typically positioned sitting up or supine with the leg internally rotated, depending on patient preference and the joint to be injected
Technique	Mark out appropriate anatomy. Use of an image intensifier is necessary to ensure needle placement. The medial and lateral gutters are preferred entry sites to minimize trauma to the anterior group's tendons and artery See Fig. 11.7
Comments	Not recommended for the novice injector

FIGURE 11.7
The ankle joint.

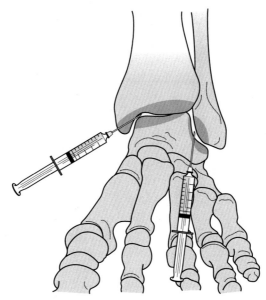

REFERENCES

Adler, R.S., Sofka, C.M., 2003. Percutaneous ultrasound-guided injections in the musculoskeletal system. Ultrasound Q. 19, 3–12.

Ayral, X., 2001. Injections in the treatment of osteoarthritis. Rheumatology 15, 609–626.

Boxer, M.C., 1994. Osteoarthritis involving the metatarsophalangeal joints and management of metatarsophalangeal joint via injection therapy. Clin. Pod. Med. Surg. 11, 125–132.

Gossec, L., Dougados, M., 2006. Do intra-articular therapies work and who will benefit most? Rheumatology 20, 131–144.

Hussain, S., Durve, R., Brennan, S., et al., 2007. The chemical stability of admixtures of injectable corticosteroid and local anaesthetics. CME Orthopaedics 4 (3), 81–83.

Khoury, N.J., El-Khoury, G.Y., Saltzman, C.L., 1996. Intraarticular foot and ankle injections to identify source of pain before arthrodesis. Am. J. Roentgenol. 167, 669–673.

Lavelle, W., Lavelle, E.D., Lavelle, L., 2007. Intra-articular injections. Anesthesiol. Clin. 25, 853–862.

Lucas, P.E., Hurwitz, S.R., Kaplan, P.A., Dussault, R.G., Maurer, E.J., 1997. Fluoroscopically-guided injections to the foot and ankle: localisation of the source of pain as a guide to treatment. Prospective study. Radiology 2042, 411–415.

McMinn, 2004. Colour Atlas of Foot and Ankle Anatomy (3rd Ed), Fig. 6.94.

McMinn, 2004. Colour Atlas of Foot and Ankle Anatomy (3rd Ed), Fig. 6.127.

Newman, J., 2003. Diagnostic and therapeutic injections of the foot and ankle. Semin. Roentgenol. 39, 85–94.

Saifuddin, A., Abdus-Samee, M., Mann, C., et al., 2005. CT guided diagnostic foot injections. Clin. Radiol. 60, 191–195.

Saunders and Longworth, 2006. Injection Techniques in Orthopaedics and Sports Medicine, pg. 137.

Solan, M.C., Calder, J.D.F., Bendall, S.P., 2001. Manipulation and injection for hallux rigidus. J. Bone Joint Surg. 83B, 706–708.

Tallia, A.F., Cardone, D.A., 2003. Diagnostic and therapeutic injection of the foot and ankle. Am. Fam. Physician 68, 1356–1362.

Vanore, J.V., Christensen, J.C., Kravitz, S.R., et al., 2003. Diagnosis and treatment of first metatarsophalangeal joint disorders. Section 2: hallux rigidus. J. Foot Ankle Surg. 42, 124–136.

Ward, S.T., Williams, P.L., Purkayastha, S., 2008. Intra-articular corticosteroid injections in the foot and ankle: a prospective 1-year follow-up investigation. J. Foot Ankle Surg. 47, 138–144.

BIBLIOGRAPHY AND FURTHER READING

Cahill, A.M., Cho, S.S., Baskin, K.M., et al., 2007. Benefit of fluoroscopically guided intra-articular long-acting corticosteroid injection for subtalar arthritis in juvenile idiopathic arthritis. Pediatr. Radiol. 37, 544–548.

Charalambous, C.P., Tryfonidis, M., Sadiq, S., et al., 2003. Septic arthritis following intra-articular steroid injection of the knee: a survey of current practice regarding antiseptic technique used during intra-articular injection of the knee. Clin. Rheumatol. 22, 386–390.

Cheng, J., Salahadin, A., 2007. Complications of joint, tendon, and muscle injections. Tech. Reg. Anesth. Pain Manag. 11, 141–147.

Chow, E., 1998. Diagnostic and therapeutic foot and ankle injections. Semin. Musculoskelet. Radiol. 24, 421–432.

Cleary, A.G., Murphy, H.D., Davidson, J.E., 2003. Intra-articular corticosteroid injections in juvenile idiopathic arthritis. Arch. Dis. Childhood 88, 192–196.

Courtney, P., Doherty, M., 2005. Joint aspiration and injection. Rheumatology 19, 345–369.

Creamer, P., 1997. Intra-articular corticosteroid injections in osteoarthritis: do they work and if so, how? Ann. Rheum. Dis. 56, 634–636.

Dacre, J.E., Beeney, N., Scott, D.L., 1989. Injections and physiotherapy for the painful stiff shoulder. Ann. Rheum. Dis. 48 (4), 322–325.

De Smeta, A.A., 2004. Ultrasound-guided injections and aspirations of the extremities. Semin. Roentgenol. 39, 145–154.

Dooley, P., Martin, R., 2002. Corticosteroid injections and arthrocentesis. Can. Fam. Physician 48, 285–292.

Fadale, P.D., Wiggins, M.D., 1994. Corticosteroid injections: their use and abuse. J. Am. Acad. Orthop. Surg. 2, 133–140.

Genovese, M.C., 1998. Joint and soft-tissue injection. A useful adjuvant to systemic and local treatment. Postgrad. Med. 103 (2), 125–134.

Gray, R.G., Tenenbaum, J., Gottlieb, N.L., 1981. Local corticosteroid injection treatment in rheumatic disorders. Semin. Arthritis Rheum. 10, 231–254.

Hall, S., Buchbinder, R., 2004. Do imaging methods that guide needle placement improve outcome? Ann. Rheum. Dis. 63, 1007–1008.

Haslock, I., MacFarlane, D., Speed, C., 1995. Intra-articular and soft tissue injections: a survey of current practice. Br. J. Rheumatol. 34, 449–452.

Hill Jr., J.J., Trapp, R., Colliver, J., 1989. Survey on the use of corticosteroid injections by orthopaedists. Contemp. Orthop. 18, 39–45.

Jacobs, L.G., Barton, M.A., Wallace, W.A., Ferrousis, J., Dunn, N.A., Bossingham, D.H., 1991. Intra-articular distension and steroids in the management of capsulitis of the shoulder. Br. Med. J. 302 (6791), 1498–1501.

Jones, A., Regan, M., Ledingham, J., et al., 1993. Importance of placement of intra-articular steroid injections. BMJ 307, 1329–1330.

Jones, D.M., Saltzman, C.L., El-Khoury, G., 1999. The diagnosis of the os trigonum syndrome with a fluoroscopically controlled injection of local anaesthetic. Iowa Orthopaed. J. 19, 122–126.

Kumar, N., Newman, R.J., 1999. Complications of intra- and peri-articular steroid injections. Br. J. Gen. Pract. 49, 465–466.

Lento, P.H., Primack, S., 2008. Advances and utility of diagnostic ultrasound in musculoskeletal medicine. Curr. Rev. Musculoskel. Med. 1, 24–31.

Noerdlinger, M.A., Fadale, P.D., 2001. The role of injectable corticosteroids in orthopedics. Orthopedics 24, 400–405.

Rifat, S.F., Moeller, J.L., 2001. Basics of joint injection: general techniques and tips for safe, effective use. Postgrad. Med. 109 (1), 157–160, 165–166.

Rifat, S.F., Moeller, J.L., 2001. Site-specific techniques of joint injection. Useful additions to your treatment repertoire. Postgrad. Med. 109 (3), 129–130, 135–136.

Rizk, T.E., Pinals, R.S., Talaiver, A.S., 1991. Corticosteroid injections in adhesive capsulitis: investigation of their value and site. Arch Phys. Med. Rehabil. 72 (1), 20–22.

Rosenberg, J.N., 2001. Corticosteroid injections of joints and soft tissues. Available at: http://www.emedicine.com/pmr/topic211.htm (accessed 22 Jan 2005).

Sami, F., Rifat, M.D., Moeller, J.L., 2001. Postgrad. Med. 109 (1), http://www.postgradmed.com/issues/2001/01_01/rifat.htm (accessed 4 Dec 2005).

Saunders, S., Longworth, S., 2006. Injection Techniques in Orthopaedics and Sports Medicine: A Practical Manual for Doctors and Physiotherapists, third ed. Elsevier, Edinburgh.

Silver, T., 2007. Joint and Soft Tissue Injection: Injecting with Confidence, fourth ed. Radcliffe Publishing, Oxon.

Sparling, M., Malleson, P., Wood, B., Petty, R. 1990. Radiographic followup of joints injected with triamcinolone hexacetonide for the management of childhood arthritis. Arthritis Rheum. 33 (6), 821–826.

von Essen, R., Savolainen, H.A., 1989. Bacterial infection following intra-articular injection. A brief review. Scand. J. Rheumatol. 18(1), 7–12.

Weiss, J.J., Ting, Y.M., 1978. Arthrography-assisted intra-articular injection of steroids in treatment of adhesive capsulitis. Arch. Phys. Med. Rehabil. 59 (6), 285–287.

COMMON FOOT AND ANKLE CONDITIONS: SOFT TISSUE INJECTIONS

12

GENERAL CONSIDERATIONS

A guide to soft tissue injection is presented below with further examples included on the accompanying DVD to the book.

Injection therapy for plantar fasciitis and plantar digital neuritis is common practice. The use of corticosteroid injection therapies in tendonopathies – especially with regard to the potential for rupture – is particularly controversial; however their use is certainly reported widely in the literature. For example, Jones (1985) postulates that many cases of tendon pain are caused by a partial rupture of the tendon and that this becomes complete regardless of whether local steroid has been injected or not. The role of inflammation in tendinitis is the subject of debate, and many authors prefer the terms "tendinosis" or "tendinopathy" to describe the pathological changes within the tendon (Khan et al. 1999). Paavola et al. (2002) note that although a complete tendon rupture after steroid injection has been reported, no reliable proof exists of the deleterious effects of peritendinous injections and state that conclusions in the literature are based on uncontrolled case reports that fail under scientific scrutiny. Hayes et al. (2000) are also of the opinion that the issue of corticosteroids and their effect on the healing of tendon pathology has not been addressed sufficiently or answered adequately. Few studies have used a well-controlled injury model. They note that steroid dosage and selection also appear to be random but that their experience – in conjunction with a complete review of the literature – leads them to believe that the use of local corticosteroid injection is a valid treatment option. They go on to state that the use of local corticosteroid injection for the treatment of tendonopathy, with the exception of the Achilles' tendon, is not only an option, but an effective means of therapy. In contrast, Da Cruz (1988) reported on a prospective, randomized, double-blind study of 28 patients presenting with Achilles paratendonitis injected with a peritendonous injection of either methyl prednisolone acetate in 0.25% Marcain or 2 mL of 0.25% Marcain alone. His results indicated that peritendonous injection of methyl prednisolone acetate is of no value in Achilles paratendonitis.

In summary, the relevance of the steroid used, the tissue affected, the extent of the tendon problem, the duration of the symptoms, the phase of healing at the time of injections, and the post injection events – especially loading – remain undetermined.

HEEL PAIN

Thomas et al. (2001) state that mechanical factors are the most common aetiology of heel pain. Other causes include traumatic, neurological, arthritic, infectious, neoplastic, autoimmune, and other systemic conditions (Fig. 12.1).

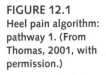

FIGURE 12.1
Heel pain algorithm: pathway 1. (From Thomas, 2001, with permission.)

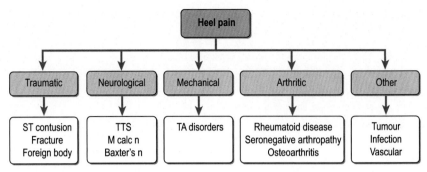

PLANTAR FASCIITIS

See Table 12.1 and Fig. 12.2 for plantar fasciitis.

Table 12.1 Plantar fasciitis

Anatomy	The insertion of a tendon or a ligament into a bone is called the enthesis. The plantar fascia (aka plantar aponeurosis) is a thickened, fibrous connective tissue structure that originates from the medial tubercle of the calcaneus and runs forward to insert in the transverse metatarsal ligament and proximal phalanges. It is made up of predominantly longitudinally oriented collagen fibres The function of the plantar fascia is to: • Prevent medial longitudinal arch collapse. • Aid purchase of the hallux in propulsion • Assist in resupination of the subtalar joint (STJ) during propulsion • Assist the posterior compartment muscles by limiting STJ pronation during standing and walking
Pathology	Plantar fasciitis is the most common cause of heel pain Definition: insertional heel pain of the plantar fascia with or without the presence of a heel spur (Thomas et al. 2001) The condition is generally seen in the adult population. Patients present with plantar heel pain on weight-bearing, either first thing in the morning or upon arising or after sitting for a period of rest (poststatic dyskinesia). The pain tends to decrease after a few minutes then returns over the course of the day as the time on the foot increases. Associated findings may include high body mass index, tightness of the Achilles' tendon, prolonged standing, and inappropriate shoe wear. The clinician is usually able to palpate pain on the plantar medial heel. Most authors cite mechanical plantar fasciitis resulting from repeated microtrauma due to overuse, which results in microtears of the tissue substance until a macroinjury occurs. Recent papers have termed the condition a fasciosis rather than fasciitis to delineate that the condition is not an inflammatory disorder. The diagnosis is a clinical one in the majority of cases. Radiographs are of limited value A heel spur is seen in 10–15% of the normal population but in 50–75% of those with heel pain. If present, it is usually superior to the PF in the flexor digitorum brevis attachment (McCarthy–Gorecki 1979). Subcalcaneal heel spurs are therefore not traction spurs, as commonly believed, as they do not develop within the plantar fascia itself. Kumai–Benjamin (2002) suggest instead that they develop as a consequence of degenerative changes that occur in the plantar fascia enthesis

Table 12.1 Plantar fasciitis—cont'd

Treatment	It is not uncommon for patients to be injected on first presentation of this condition. It is certainly the authors' experience that this is often the first-line treatment offered by general practitioners in the UK. The American College of Foot & Ankle Surgery Guidelines for Heel Pain (2001) strongly suggest a stepwise approach to treatment. First-line treatment should therefore be conservative in nature using the RICE (rest, ice, compression, elevation) system, judicious use of NSAIDs, heel cushioning, orthotics, and strapping. Do not use injection therapy until these treatments have been tried and have failed or are only partially successful
	Phase 1: • Rest, ice, compression, and elevation • Stretching • NSAIDs, arch pads/heel cushions, taping, weight loss if appropriate Phase 2, if no improvement after 6 weeks: • Continue initial therapy • Prescription orthotics, night splints, CAM walker • **Steroid injections – see below** Phase 3, if no improvement 4–6 months after initial treatment: • Continue initial therapy • Below knee cast • Shockwave therapy (ESWT) • Surgery
Equipment	2.5 or 5 mL syringe 25 mm (1 inch) 23 gauge (blue) needle
Drug(s)	40 mg of methylprednisolone mixed with local anaesthetic
Positioning	The patient is positioned sitting up or supine, depending on patient preference. Note: this can be a painful injection for the patient
Technique (SEE VIDEO 15)	Mark the area that is the most painful to palpation and visualize where the plantar fascia is in relation to this mark. Note that this is not the usual site of a bony heel spur, which, if present, is normally superior to the plantar fascia in the origin of the intrinsic musculature
	Different approaches have been described in the literature. The potential advantage of the direct plantar approach is that, in theory, it should be easier to find the tender spot as you are injecting directly over and into it; however, the disadvantage is the increased pain at the injection site. The medial approach is slightly less painful for the patient than the plantar approach and therefore the technique we recommend. Advance the needle deeper laterally to correspond with the skin marking. Start superficially and move deeper (withdraw slightly then re-angle more deeply) in a sequential manner until positive feedback from the tip of the needle is elicited. Look for the maximum point of tenderness to deposit the steroid. Taking this approach minimizes the chance of damage to the nerve – although the medial plantar nerve is deeper than the maximum point of tenderness, there are reports in the literature that point to accidental nerve damage following injections for plantar fasciitis (Snow et al. 2005). Inject as either a bolus or peppering technique

Continued

Table 12.1 Plantar fasciitis—cont'd

Comments	The evidence base for injecting plantar fasciitis with corticosteroids is somewhat controversial. None the less, injection therapy is performed by many practitioners in different professional disciplines and is one of the more common infiltrations that will be performed in the foot. The management of this condition via injection therapy is a book in itself. Crawford (1999) points to the limited usefulness of steroid in the management of the condition, pointing out that plantar fasciitis represents more of a fasciosis rather than a true fasciitis. Fascial rupture has been noted (Acevedo & Beskin 1998) which can be difficult to treat. Fortunately rupture is rare but if the clinician is in any doubt ordering an MRI is helpful to exclude this before injections are performed. Rupture in itself could not be considered negligent as surgery creates a deliberate rupture

FIGURE 12.2
Plantar fasciitis.

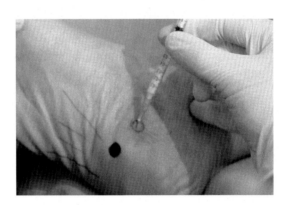

PLANTAR CALCANEAL BURSITIS

See Table 12.2 for plantar calcaneal bursitis.

Table 12.2 Plantar calcaneal bursitis

Anatomy	The plantar surface of the calcaneus presents a roughened appearance. The plantar heel pad is a specialized organisation of tissue that lies on the plantar aspect of this bone. Cylinders of fat separated by small septa form an integral network which is arranged in a precise fashion and serves as a shock absorber for the bottom of the heel
Pathology	Plantar calcaneal bursitis is inflammation of the adventitious bursa beneath the plantar aspect of the calcaneal tuberosity. It is associated with shearing stress due to an altered angle of heel strike Clinical features: • Increasingly severe burning, aching, throbbing pain on the plantar surface of the heel • There is usually a history of increased activity/weight gain • The heel will seem normal but may feel warm • Direct compression causes pain
Treatment	Initial treatment is centred on reduction of compressive and shearing forces to the plantar heel pad. Injection therapy is indicated in recalcitrant cases

Table 12.2 Plantar calcaneal bursitis—cont'd

Equipment	2.5 or 5 mL syringe 25 mm (1 inch) 23 gauge (blue) needle
Drug(s)	40 mg of methylprednisolone mixed with local anaesthetic
Positioning	The patient is positioned sitting up or supine, depending on patient preference
Technique (SEE VIDEO 16)	Direct infiltration into the point of maximal tenderness Inject as either a bolus or peppering technique Note: this can be a painful injection for the patient
Comments	Use concurrent heel cushioning

TARSAL TUNNEL SYNDROME

See Table 12.3 and Fig. 12.3 for tarsal tunnel syndrome.

Table 12.3 Tarsal tunnel syndrome

Anatomy	The *tarsal canal* is located behind and under the medial malleolus and becomes the *tarsal tunnel* as a result of the flexor retinaculum (laciniate ligament) passing over and creating a closed space. The flexor retinaculum blends with the plantar fascia and is therefore affected by the tension on the plantar fascia since both are anchored at the calcaneus and connected to each other. Four fibrous septa emerge from the interior surface of the flexor retinaculum. The third channel, counting from medial to lateral, contains the nerve and vascular structures. The (bifurcated) nerve enters the foot at the abductor canal, traditionally referred to as the porta pedis
Pathology	Tension on the plantar fascia (e.g. in pronation) may affect the tension on the retinaculum and alter the volume of the tunnel. Tarsal tunnel syndrome describes an entrapment or compressional neuropathy of the tibial nerve in the posterior medial compartment of the foot. The fascia of the abductor hallucis helps form this portal and hypertrophy of this muscle may also put greater pressure on the nerve
	An entrapment neuropathy is a focal neuropathy caused by mechanical impingement at a vulnerable anatomical site. A compressive neuropathy is one in which there is damage to a peripheral nerve by pressure. The symptoms and signs of an entrapment or compressive neuropathy may be motor, sensory, autonomic or mixed. Authors suggest that constriction of the porta pedis may be as influential in producing symptoms. Other causes include space-occupying lesions, nerve tumours, bony exostoses and variscosites. Signs and symptoms include paresthesia in the sole of the foot and Tinel's sign or Valleix's phenomenon elicited by tapping (percussing) of the course of the nerve. A positive outcome may be seen with diagnostic nerve conduction studies

Treatment	Identify the aetiology and consider judicious use of:
	  • NSAIDs
	  • Strapping
	  • Physical therapy
	  • Orthotics
	  • Mobilization
	  • **Steroid therapy**
	Use of steroid injection, must, as always, only be used as part of an overall treatment plan and is also used with respect to the underlying cause. For instance, tarsal tunnel can present secondary to hyperpronation or trauma and the underlying cause should always be addressed where possible

Continued

Table 12.3 Tarsal tunnel syndrome—cont'd

Equipment	2.5 or 5 mL syringe 25 mm (1 inch) 23 gauge (blue) needle
Drug(s)	40 mg of methylprednisolone mixed with local anaesthetic
Positioning	The patient is positioned sitting up or supine, depending on patient preference
Technique	Typically there is a point of maximum tenderness. Author preference is for 30–40 mg of methylprednisolone injected into the point of maximum tenderness. Visualize the course of the posterior tibial tendon, which should be avoided
Comments	Warn the patient that they will develop numbness in the plantar foot

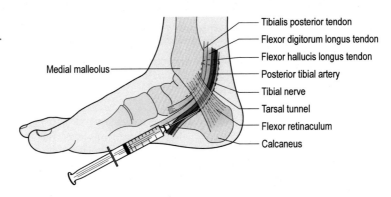

FIGURE 12.3
Tarsal tunnel syndrome.
(After McMinn, 2004,
with permission.)

Medial malleolus

Tibialis posterior tendon
Flexor digitorum longus tendon
Flexor hallucis longus tendon
Posterior tibial artery
Tibial nerve
Tarsal tunnel
Flexor retinaculum
Calcaneus

MORTON'S NEUROMA

See Table 12.4 and Fig. 12.4 for Morton's neuroma.

Table 12.4 Plantar digital neuritis

Anatomy	The common digital nerves originate from the medial and lateral plantar nerves. The medial plantar nerve divides into many branches, including the medial three common digital nerves, which bifurcate to supply cutaneous branches to the medial three-and-a-half digits. The lateral plantar nerve gives rise to two common digital nerves, supplying cutaneous branches to the lateral one-and-a-half digits. Branches from the medial and lateral plantar nerves unite around the third intermetatarsal space. As the common digital nerves travel distally, they pass deep to the transverse intermetatarsal ligament. The angulation of the nerve is most marked when the toes are hyperextended at the metatarsal phalangeal joints; plantar flexion decreases the pressure
Pathology	Plantar digital neuritis, aka intermetatarsal neuroma or Morton's neuroma, is an entrapment neuropathy of a common digital nerve and is a common forefoot complaint. Larson et al. (2005) call for the diagnosis of nerve compression to be further distinguished by naming the involved nerve rather than using eponymous terms as, confusingly, entrapment of the 1st to the 5th nerves has been reported by Joplin, Hauser, Heuter, Morton and Islen

Table 12.4 Plantar digital neuritis—cont'd

	Histologically, a painful fusiform swelling of the nerve develops, marked by perineural fibrosis of the nerve caused by repetitive trauma or secondary fibrosis. Symptoms include a tingling or burning sensation that can radiate up into the toe, perhaps with sharp shooting sensations. Symptoms are worse with activity aggravated by tight shoes and relieved by removing the shoe and massaging the foot
	Although initially described by Morton in the third interspace, it is also quite commonly found in the second interspace. However, for a suspected neuroma in the second interspace, also look for signs of hyperpronation and mechanical overload as these often coexist. A mechanically induced capsulitis may cause pressure on the nerve, leading the clinician to identify a neuroma when the true cause is joint-related
	A range of diagnostic modalities are available with various papers talking about the use of MRI and ultrasound. Ultrasound is somewhat operator-dependent and in most cases the diagnosis of a neuroma can be made on a clinical presentation only. The site of the entrapment is usually distal to the metatarsal heads and is often between the bases of the proximal phalanges. The clinician should therefore look for point tenderness between and anterior to adjacent metatarsal head/phalanges and not be surprised to find that the point of pain is somewhat more distal than often thought. The Mulder's click and lateral squeeze tests are commonly performed tests but in our experience, the patient's description of the pain, and site of point tenderness plantarly, are the best indications of a diagnosis. Also consider the digital stretch test recently described by Cloke and Greiss (2006)
Treatment	Padding and orthoses can be useful in early presentations of the condition. Where shoe gear is implicated, advise accordingly The authors' second-line treatment is a course of steroid therapy but sclerosing alcohol injections (see Chapter 13) can also be employed. Surgical excision is considered in recalcitrant cases
Equipment	2.5 or 5 mL syringe 25 mm (1 inch) 23 gauge (blue) needle
Drug(s)	40 mg of methylprednisolone mixed with local anaesthetic
Positioning	The patient is positioned sitting up or supine, depending on patient preference
Technique (SEE VIDEO 17)	It is very useful to mark the foot up anatomically in the first few times that you perform this injection. Mark the metatarsal heads and the base of the proximal phalanges and visualize how distal the point of pain usually is. These are best injected from a dorsal approach, angling the needle at 90° and gently advancing the needle from the dorsal to the plantar surface of the foot to where the neuroma lies. Often, resistance from the deep transverse metatarsal ligament can be found on advancing the needle. It is imperative to grasp the syringe very lightly between the thumb and forefinger as, on occasion, the needle tip will touch the neuroma directly. This can cause the patient to jump and if the syringe is being gripped too tightly, the patient and/or the operator may suffer a needle stick injury. It is therefore worth gently probing with the tip of the needle to locate a tender spot. When the point of tenderness is found the steroid can be infiltrated. Aspiration is a best practice though it would be very difficult to give a significant intravascular dose due to the small cross-sectional diameter of the arteries and veins at this point. Be aware that if the needle is advanced too far plantarly then the patient may feel pricking of the skin from the inside, and what is thought of as feedback is merely pain from the inside of the skin.
Comments	If available, injecting with ultrasound (US) guidance is ideal for needle tip placement. US will also identify intermetatarsal bursae

FIGURE 12.4
Morton's neuroma.

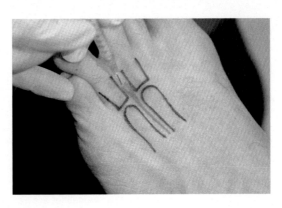

PRE-ACHILLES BURSITIS AND HAGLUND'S DEFORMITY

See Table 12.5 and Fig. 12.5 for pre-Achilles bursitis and Haglund's deformity.

Table 12.5 Pre-Achilles bursitis and Haglund's deformity

Anatomy	The posterior aspect of the calcaneus is divided into 3 areas. The upper surface is smooth and separated from the tendo Achilles by the only anatomical bursa in the foot – the pre-Achilles bursa – and fatty tissue. The middle area is rough and has a ridge that gives attachment to the tendo Achilles. The lower area is the weight-bearing surface and slopes downwards and forwards
Pathology	Thomas et al. (2001) categorize posterior heel pathology as: • Insertional Achilles tendinitis • Bursitis (adventitious) often associated with Haglund's deformity Patrick Haglund was the first to describe a deformity associated with pain to the back of the heel in 1928. He identified pain associated with bony prominence to the posterior superiolateral aspect of the calcaneus. Some clinicians refer to any enlargement of the posterior heel as Haglund's deformity but the distinction should be made between the true Haglund exostosis, which is posterior superiolateral, and a retro calcaneal exostosis. An adventitious bursa may also form over the retro calcaneal exostosis. The pre-Achilles bursa may also become inflamed
Treatment	Padding and orthoses can be useful in early presentations of these conditions. Where shoe gear is implicated, advise accordingly Where a true bursitis exists, the authors' second-line treatment is a diagnostic block of local anaesthetic followed by a small dose of steroid
Equipment	2.5 or 5 mL syringe 25 mm (1 inch) 23 gauge (blue) needle
Drug(s)	20 mg of methylprednisolone mixed with local anaesthetic
Positioning	The patient is typically on their side or prone, depending on patient preference
Technique	Inject from the lateral side into the pre-Achilles bursa, avoiding the tendon
Comments	The posterior heel is the second most common location of mechanically induced symptoms

FIGURE 12.5
Pre-Achilles bursitis and Haglund's deformity.
(After McMinn, 2004, with permission.)

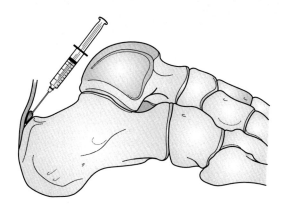

TENDON PATHOLOGY

See Table 12.6 and Fig. 12.6 for tendon pathology.

Table 12.6 Tendon pathology

Anatomy	Tendons, the fibrous ends of muscles by which they are attached to bones, vary considerably. Usually the origin of the muscle is the fixed point and the insertion the movable point. Generally, the tendons are well developed at their insertions and relatively stronger than the muscle to which they are attached. In sudden trauma the muscle belly or the tendon attachment is more liable to damage than the tendon itself. Tendons are composed of fascicles of collagen fibres running parallel to the long axis of the tendon. They extend very little but are relatively flexible and are able to curve around bony surfaces, e.g., peroneus longus around the cuboid bone. They have a poor vascular network so appear white. They can take the form of: (a) Round as in tendons of fingers and toes (b) Oval as in the tendo Achilles (c) Flattened as in the plantaris or the patella tendons
Pathology	Tendonitis or tendonopathy of the tendons around the ankle is increasingly being seen in orthopaedic, musculoskeletal, and podiatry clinics. Achilles tendonopathy and posterior tibialis tendon dysfunction (PTTD) are common and these foot pathologies are themselves the subject of much literature and debate The vast majority of injuries to the TA involve a disruption of the tendon architecture. The usual area of rupture or weakness is at the point of poorest blood supply – 2 to 6 cm proximal to its calcaneal insertion; rupture at the myo-tendinous or tendo-osseous junctions occurs much less frequently. As with PTTD, it is believed that there is almost always some degenerative process at the site of rupture
Treatment	Mechanical problems often are eliminated by: • Stretching exercises • Custom orthoses to alleviate overpronation if present • Stretching • Cross-training Injection therapy may be considered prior to surgical intervention The authors' recommendation is to avoid the use of stronger steroids such as triamcinolone in tendon pathology and to start with weaker or soluble solutions such as hydrocortisone or betamethasone. Use these in low doses combined with a higher ratio of local anaesthesia. In effect it is a diagnostic local anaesthetic approach combined with a small amount of steroid to try to get a small therapeutic effect

Continued

Table 12.6 Tendon pathology—cont'd

Equipment	2.5 or 5 mL syringe 25 mm (1 inch) 23 gauge (blue) needle
Drug(s)	20–40 mg, depending on the tendon, of hydrocortisone methylprednisolone mixed with local anaesthetic
Positioning	The patient is typically on their side or prone, depending on patient preference
Technique	Follow the course of the tendon and keep the needle within the tendon sheath. Do not inject into the body of the tendon. If you are able to, then it suggests that the tendons have internal lytic or mucoid degeneration
Comments	Proceed with caution around tendons! Readers are directed to a new technique of high-volume image-guided injections in chronic Achilles tendinopathy published by Chan and colleagues in 2008. In our personal communication with the authors we feel that this approach may provide an advantage over previous injection techniques

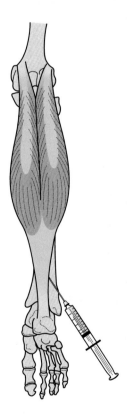

FIGURE 12.6
Tendon pathology.

REFERENCES

Acevedo, J.I., Beskin, J.L., 1998. Complications of plantar fascial rupture associated with steroid injection. Foot Ankle Int. 19, 91–97.

Cloke, D.J., Greiss, M.E., 2006. The digital nerve stretch test: a sensitive indicator of Morton's neuroma and neuritis. J. Foot Ankle Surg. 12 (4), 201–203.

Crawford, F., Atkins, D., Young, P., Edwards, J., 1999. Steroid injection for heel pain: evidence of short-term effectiveness. A randomized controlled trial. Rheumatology 38, 974–977.

DaCruz, D.J., 1988. Achilles paratendonitis: an evaluation of steroid injection. Br. J. Sports Med. 22 (2), 64–65.

Haglund, P., 1928. Beitrag zur Kinik der Achillesscehne. Aschr-Orthop. Chir. 49, 49.

Hayes Jr., D.W., Gilbertson, E.K., Mandracchia, V.J., Dolphin, T.F., 2000. Tendon pathology in the foot: the use of corticosteroid injection therapy. Clin. J. Pod. Med. Surg. 17 (4), 723–735.

Jones, J.G., 1985. Achilles tendon rupture following steroid injection. J. Bone Joint Surg. Am. 67, 170.

Khan, K.M., Cook, J.L., Bonar, F., et al., 1999. Histopathology of common tendinopathies. Sports Med. 27 (6), 393–408.

Larson, E.E., Barrett, S.L., Battiston, B., Maloney Jr., C.T., Dellon, A.L., 2005. Accurate nomenclature for forefoot nerve entrapment: a historical perspective. J. Am. Podiatr. Med. Assoc. 95 (3), 298–306.

Paavola, M., Kannus, P., Jarvinen, T.A., et al., 2002. Treatment of tendon disorders. Is there a role for corticosteroid injection. Foot Ankle Clin. 7 (3), 501–513.

Thomas, D.P.M., Christensen, J.C., Kravitz, S.R., 2001. The Diagnosis and Treatment of Heel Pain Clinical Practice Guideline Heel Pain Panel.

Thomas, J.L., et al., 2001. The diagnosis and treatment of heel pain. J. Foot Ankle Surg. 40, 329–340.

BIBLIOGRAPHY AND FURTHER READING

Adler, R.S., Sofka, C.M., 2003. Percutaneous ultrasound-guided injections in the musculoskeletal system. Ultrasound Q. 19, 3–12.

Aldridge, T., 2004. Diagnosing heel pain in adults. Am. Fam. Physician 70, 332–338.

Assendelft, W.J., Hay, E.M., Adhead, R., Bouter, L.M., 1996. Corticosteroid injections for lateral epicondylitis: a systematic overview. Br. J. Gen. Pract. 46, 209–216.

Atkins, D., Crawford, F., Edwards, J., 1999. A systematic review of treatments for the painful heel. Rheumatology 38, 968–973.

Baravarian, B., Rhim, B., 2007. A new algorithm for treating plantar fasciitis. Podiatry Today 20 (11), 84–89.

Barrett, S.J., 2006. Should you change your approach to plantar fasciosis? Podiatry Today 19, 48–56.

Barrett, S.J., O'Malley, R., 1999. Plantar fasciitis and other causes of heel pain. Am. Fam. Physician 59, 2200–2206.

Baxter, D.E., Thigpen, C.M., 1984. Heel pain: operative results. Foot Ankle 5, 16.

Bertouch, J., 2002. Corticosteroid injection for plantar fasciitis. Medicine Today 3, 112.

Blockey, N.J., 1956. The painful heel – a controlled trial of the value of hydrocortisone. Br. Med. J. 2, 1277–1278.

Boberg, J.S., Dauphinée, D.M., 2001. Heel pain. In: Banks, A.S., Downey, M.S., Martin, D.E., Miller, S.J. (Eds.), McGlamary's Comprehensive Textbook of Foot & Ankle Surgery, third ed. Lippincott, Williams & Wilkins, Philadelphia, pp. 464–478.

Brophy, D.P., Cunnane, G., Fitzgerald, O., Gibney, R.G., 1995. Technical report: ultrasound guidance for injection of soft tissue lesions around the heel in chronic inflammatory arthritis. Clin. Radiol. 50, 120–122.

Buccelli, T.A., Hall, H.R., Solmen, J.D., 2005. Sterile abscess formation following a corticosteroid injection for the treatment of plantar fasciitis. J. Foot Ankle Surg. 44, 466–468.

Chan, O., O'Dowd, D., Padhiar, N., et al, 2008. High volume image guided injections in chronic Achilles tendinopathy. Disabil. Rehabil. 30, 1697–1708.

Cheng, J., Abdi, S., 2007. Complications of joint, tendon, and muscle injections. Tech. Reg. Anesth. Pain Manag. 11, 141–147.

Cheng, J., Salahadin, A., 2007. Complications of joint, tendon, and muscle injections. Tech. Reg. Anesth. Pain Manag. 11, 141–147.

Cole, C., Seto, C., Gazewood, J., 2005. Plantar fasciitis: evidence-based review of diagnosis and therapy. Am. Fam. Physician 72, 2237–2242.

Conti, R.J., Shinder, M., 1991. Soft tissue calcifications induced by local corticosteroid injection. J. Foot Surg. 30, 34–37.

Cooper, A.J., Mize, M.S., 2007. Comparison of MRI and local anesthetic tendon sheath injection in the diagnosis of posterior tibial tendon tenosynovitis. Foot Ankle Int. 28 (11).

Crawford, F., Thomson, C., 2004. Interventions for treating plantar heel pain. Cochrane Database of Syst. Rev. Issue 3. John Wiley and Sons, Chichester.

DaCruz, D.J., Geeson, M., Allen, M.J., Phair, I., 1988. Achilles paratendonitis: an evaluation of steroid injection. Br. J. Sports Med. 22, 64–65.

Dagenai, S., Haldeman, D.C., Wooley, J.R., 2005. Intraligamentous injection of sclerosing solutions (prolotherapy) for spinal pain: a critical review of the literature. Spine J. 5, 310–328.

Dasgupta, B., Bowles, J., 1995. Scintigraphic localisation of steroid injection site in plantar fasciitis. Lancet 346, 1400–1401.

Dockery, G.L., 2002. When injection therapy can help relieve painful lesions. Podiatry Today 15 (6), 30–36.

Frater, C., Vu, D., van der Wall, H., Perera, C., et al., 2006. Bone scintigraphy predicts outcome of steroid injection for plantar fasciitis. J. Nucl. Med. 47, 1577–1580.

Genc, H., Saracoglu, M., Nacir, B., et al., 2005. Long-term ultrasonography follow-up of plantar fasciitis patients treated with steroid injections. Joint Bone Spine 72, 61–65.

Gidumal, R., Evanski, P., 1985. Calcaneal osteomyelitis following steroid injection: a case report. Foot Ankle 6, 44–46.

Gill, S.S., Gelbke, M.K., Mattson, S.L., et al., 2004. Fluoroscopically guided low-volume peritendinous corticosteroid injection for Achilles tendonopathy. J. Bone Joint Surg. Am. 86, 802–806.

Gruber, H., Kovacs, P., Peer, S., Frischhut, B., Bodner, G., 2004. Sonographically guided phenol injection in painful stump neuroma. Am. J. Roentgenol. 182, 952–954.

Haslock, I., MacFarlane, D., Speed, C., Intra-articular and soft tissue injections: a survey of current practice. Br. J. Rheumatol. 34, 449–452.

Henricson, A.S., Westlin, N.E., 1984. Chronic calcaneal pain in athletes: entrapment of the calcaneal nerve? Am. J. Sports Med. 12, 152.

Imberman, N., 1990. Treatment of Morton's neuroma. J. Am. Podiatr. Med. Assoc. 80, 47.

Kamel, M., Kotob, H., 2000. High frequency ultrasonographic findings in plantar fasciitis and assessment of local steroid injection. J. Rheumatol. 27, 2139–2141.

Kane, D., Greaney, T., Bresnihan, B., et al., 1998. Ultrasound guided injection of recalcitrant plantar fasciitis. Ann. Rheum. Dis. 57, 383–384.

Kenzora, J.E., 1987. The painful heel syndrome: an entrapment neuropathy. Bull. Hosp. Jt. Dis. 47, 178.

Khan, K.M., 2002. Painful, overuse tendon conditions have a non-inflammatory pathology. BMJ 324, 626–627.

Kiter, E., Çelikba, E., Akkaya, S., et al., 2006. Comparison of injection modalities in the treatment of plantar heel pain: a randomized controlled trial. JAPMA 96, 293–296.

Kriss, S., 2003. Injectable steroids in the management of heel pain. A prospective randomised trial. Br. J. Podiatry 6 (2), 40–42.

Kumai, T., Benjamin, M., 2002. Heel spur formation and the subcalcaneal enthesis of the plantar fascia. J. Rheumatol. 29, 1957–1964.

Kunihiro, Y., Kazuto, N., Atsushi, K., Moroe, B., 2005. Old ruputure of Achilles tendon following steroid injection: a case report. St. Marianna Med. J. 33 (5), 467–471.

Lapidus, P.W., Guidotti, F.P., 1959. Local injections of hydrocortisone in 495 orthopaedic patients. IMS Ind. Med. Surg. 26, 234–244.

Lapidus, P.W., Guidotti, F.P., 1987. Painful heel: report of 323 patients with 364 painful heels. Clin. Orthop. 39, 178.

Lemont, H., Ammirati, K.M., Usen, N., 2003. Plantar fasciitis: a degenerative process (fasciosis) without inflammation. JAPMA 93, 234–237.

Lucas, P.E., Hurwitz, S.R., Kaplan, P.A., et al., 1997. Flouroscopically guided injections into the foot and ankle: localization of the source of pain as a guide to treatment – prospective study. Radiology 204, 411–415.

McLaughlin, G.J., Handoll, H.H.G., 2001. Interventions for treating acute and chronic Achilles tendonitis. Cochrane Database Syst. Rev. Issue 2. John Wiley and Sons, Chichester.

McMinn, 2004. Colour Atlas of Foot and Ankle Anatomy (3rd Ed), Fig. 6.94.

McNabb, J.W., 2005. A Practical Guide to Joint and Soft Tissue Injection and Aspiration. Lippincott, Williams and Wilkins, Philadelphia.

Marshall, S., Tardif, G., Ashworth, N., 2002. Local corticosteroid injection for carpal tunnel syndrome. Cochrane Database Syst. Rev. Issue 4. John Wiley and Sons, Chichester.

Mehdizade, A., Adler, R.S., 2007. Sonographically guided flexor hallucis longus tendon sheath injection. J. Ultrasound Med. 26, 233–237.

Michelsson, J.D., 1998. Musculoskeletal Q & A. Corticosteroids for nagging heel pain. J. Med. 15 (5), 8.

Michelsson, O., Konttinen, Y.T., Paavolainen, P., Santavirta, S., 2005. Plantar heel pain and its 3-mode 4-stage treatment. Mod. Rheumatol. 15, 307–314.

Miller, R.A., Torres, J., McGuire, M., 1995. Efficacy of first-time steroid injection for painful heel syndrome. Foot Ankle Int. 16, 610–612.

Monenza, J., 2003. A guide to conservative treatment for heel pain. Podiatry Today 11, 68–76.

Newman, J.S., 2004. Diagnostic and therapeutic injections of the foot and ankle. Semin. Roentgenol. 39, 85–94.

Nimgade, A., Sullivan, M., Goldman, R., 2005. Physiotherapy, steroid injections, or rest for lateral epicondylosis? What the evidence suggests. Pain Pract. 5, 203–215.

Ogden, J., Alvarez, M.D., Cross, G.L., Jaakola, J.L., 2005. Plantar fasciotomy and orthotripsy: the effect of prior cortisone injection. Foot Ankle Int. 26, 231.

Paavola, M., Kannus, P., Järvinen, T.A.H., et al., 2002. Treatment of tendon disorders. Is there a role for corticosteroid injection. Foot Ankle Clin. N. Am. 7, 501–513.

Pigliardo, F., Briffa, N.K., Owens, J. Chronic heel pain: anatomical support for extensive tarsal tunnel release in selected cases. Br. J. Podiatry 10, 24–30.

Porter, M.D., Shadbolt, B., 2005. Intralesional corticosteroid injection versus extracorporeal shock wave therapy for plantar fasciopathy. Clin. J. Sport Med. 15, 119–124.

Pribut, S., 2007. Current approaches to the management of plantar heel pain syndrome, including the role of injectable corticosteroids. J. Am. Podiatr. Med. Assoc. 97, 68–74.

Puttaswamaiah, R., Chandran, P., 2007. Degenerative plantar fasciitis: A review of current concepts. The Foot 17, 3–9.

Rasmussen, M.R., Kitaoka, H.B., Patzer, G.L., 1996. Nonoperative treatment of plantar interdigital neuroma with a single corticosteroid injection. Clin. Orthop. Relat. Res. 326, 188–193.

Read, M.A., Motto, S.G., 1992. Tendo Achilles pain: steroids and outcome. Br. J. Sports Med. 26, 15–21.

Ritchie, D.H., 2002. Clinical podiatry. The best treatments for plantar heel pain: it's essential to review the latest outcomes studies. Podiatry Manag. 21 (6), 135–136, 138–142, 144–147.

Roberts, W.O., 1999. Plantar fascia injection. Physician Sports Med. 27 (9), 101–102.

Rome, K., 2005. Heel pain: diagnosis and management. Podiatry Now (CPD Suppl.).

Rondhuis, J.J., Huson, A., 1986. The first branch of the lateral plantar nerve and heel pain. Acta Morphol. Neerl. Scand. 24, 269.

Rosenberg, J.N., 2001. Corticosteroid injections of joints and soft tissues. http://www.emedicine.com/pmr/topic211.htm

Saragas, N.P., 2006. Hydrocortisone/local anaesthetic injection versus ultrasound in the diagnosis of interdigital neuroma. Foot Ankle Surg. 12, 149–151.

Saunders, S., Longworth, S., 2006. Injection Techniques in Orthopaedics and Sports Medicine: A Practical Manual for Doctors and Physiotherapists, third ed. Elsevier, Edinburgh.

Saygi, B., et al., 2005. Morton neuroma: comparative results of two conservative methods. Foot Ankle Int. 26, 556–559.

Schoene, L.M., 2005. A stepwise approach to treating chronic heel pain. Podiatry Today 18 (11), 58–64.

Sellman, J.R., 1994. Plantar fascial rupture associated with corticosteroid injection. Foot Ankle Int. 15, 376–381.

Shrier, I., Matheson, G.O., Kohl, H.W., 1996. Achilles tendonitis: are corticosteroid injections useful or harmful? Clin. J. Sport Med. 6, 245–250.

Silver, T., 2007. Joint and Soft Tissue Injection: Injecting with Confidence, seventh ed. Radcliffe Publishing, Oxon.

Singh, D., Angel, J., Bentley, G., Trevino, S.G., 1997. Heel pain. Br. Med. J. 315, 172–175.

Snow, D.M., Reading, J., Dalal, R., 2005. Lateral plantar nerve injury following steroid injection for plantar fasciitis. Br. J. Sports Med. 39, e41.

Sofka, C.M., Adler, R.S., 2002. Ultrasound-guided interventions in the foot and ankle. Semin. Musculoskelet. Radiol. 6, 163–168.

Sofka, C.M., Collins, A.J., Adler, R.S., 2001. Use of ultrasonographic guidance in interventional musculoskeletal procedures: a review from a single institution. J. Ultrasound Med. 20, 21–26.

Sofka, C.M., Adler, R.S., Ciavarra, G.A., Pavlov, H., 2007. Ultrasound-guided interdigital neuroma injections: short-term clinical outcomes after a single percutaneous injection: preliminary results. HSS J. 3 (1), 44–49.

Soomekh, D., Baravarian, B., 2005. Diagnostic dilemmas: how to diagnose and treat interdigital neuritis. Podiatry Today 18, 67–71.

Speed, C.A., 2001. Corticosteroid injections in tendon lesions. BMJ 323, 382–386.

Speed, C.A., 2001. Fortnightly review: corticosteriod injections in tendon lesions. BMJ 323, 382–386.

Speed, C.A., 2007. Injection therapies for soft-tissue lesions. Best Pract. Res. Clin. Rheumatol. 21, 333–347.

Stephens, M.M., Walker, G., 1997. Heel pain: an overview of its aetiology and management. Foot Ankle Surg. 3 (2), 51–60.

Stroud, C., 2002. Heel pain, plantar fasciitis, and tarsal tunnel syndrome. Curr. Opin. Orthopaed. 13, 89–92.

Tallia, A.F., Cardone, D.A., 2003. Diagnostic and therapeutic injection of the ankle and foot. Am. Fam. Physician 68, 356–362.

Thomas, A.J., Bull, M.J., Howard, A.C., Saleh, M., 1999. Peri operative ultrasound guided needle localisation of amputation stump neuroma. Injury Int. J. Care Injured 30, 689–691.

Thomas, J.L., Christensen, J.C., Kravitz, S.R., et al., 2001. The diagnosis and treatment of heel pain. J. Foot Ankle Surg. 40, 329–340.

Thomson, C.E., Gibson, J.N., Martin, D., 2004. Interventions for the treatment of Morton's neuroma. Cochrane Database Syst. Rev. 3, CD003118.

Tsai, W.C., Wang, C.L., Tang, F.T., et al., 2000. Treatment of proximal plantar fasciitis with ultrasound-guided steroid injection. Arch. Phys. Med. Rehabil. 81 (10), 1416–1421.

Vohra, P.K., Japour, C.J., 2003. Diagnostic and therapeutic management of heel pain via ultrasound-guided injection: this modality is both precise and cost-effective. Podiatry Manag. 22, 163–172.

Weil, L.S., 1994. New treatment for chronic heel pain. J. Foot Ankle Surg. 33, 216–219.

Wolgin, M., Cook, C., Graham, C., et al., 1994. Conservative treatment of plantar heel pain: long term follow-up. Foot Ankle 15, 97–102.

Young, C.C., Rutherford, D.S., Niedfeldt, M.W., 2001. Treatment of plantar fasciitis. Am. Fam. Physician 63, 467–474, 477–478.

Younger, A.S.E., Claridge, R.J., 1998. The role of diagnostic block in the management of Morton's neuroma. Can. J. Surg. 41, 127–130.

OTHER INJECTION THERAPIES

13

HYALURONIC ACID THERAPY

Hyaluronan, or hyaluronic acid (HA), is a normal vital constituent of both articular cartilage and synovial fluid. It is an unbranched high-molecular-weight polysaccharide belonging to the family of glycosaminoglycans (GAGs). It is the most abundant GAG in the human body being found in high concentrations in a variety of tissues. The largest concentration is found in the synovial fluid of joints (concentrations of between 1 and 4 mg/mL) and it is synthesized by type B synovial cells. The term "hyaluronic acid" was adopted when the biopolymer (polysaccharide) was first isolated from the vitreous of bovine eyes in 1934. The term "sodium hyaluronate" refers to the highly purified narrow-molecular-weight hyaluronans used therapeutically. A molecular schematic of hyaluronan is given in Figure 13.1.

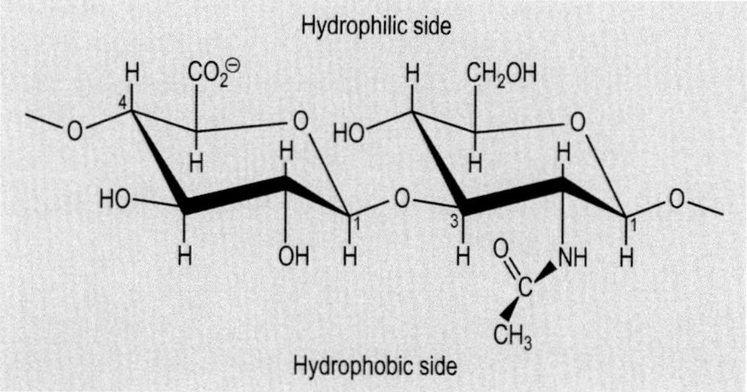

FIGURE 13.1 Hyaluronan molecular schematic. (From TRB Chemedica [UK] Ltd with permission.)

SYNOVIAL JOINTS AND THE ROLE OF HYALURONAN

As outlined in Chapter 11, synovial joints are filled with a viscous fluid called the synovial fluid, which is produced by cells of the synovial lining. The fluid can be best likened to the extracellular fluid that surrounds the body's cells. It serves a vital role in the lubrication, nutrition, and load attenuation of joints.

Role of Synovial Fluid
• Joint lubrication
• Load attenuation
• Cytoprotective
• Transport medium

Healthy synovial fluid contains 0.2–0.4% of hyaluronan with a molecular weight of between 4 and 6 million Daltons. It undergoes a constant process of production and degradation within tight homeostatic limits. Hyaluronan within the synovial fluid exhibits quite unique characteristics, possessing both viscous and elastic properties.

The viscous component, being a characteristic of liquids, confers lubricating properties to the joint. The viscosity of the synovial fluid is determined by its constituents and exhibits non-Newtonian behaviour. That is to say the viscous properties vary according to the rate of load. In the case of synovial fluid it offers greater resistance to shear at low load rates and reduced resistance at increased load rate. From a functional point of view this is important, as when joints undergo rapid movements the synovial fluid offers progressively less resistance. (Fig. 13.2).

FIGURE 13.2
Response of hyaluronan to varied load rates. (From TRB Chemedica [UK] Ltd with permission.)

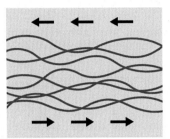

Under gradual shear stress, hyaluronan acts as a lubricant

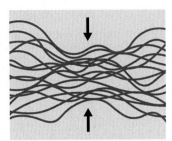

Under sudden loading, hyaluronan acts as a shock absorber

The elastic element is a characteristic of some solids and confers shock-absorbing properties to synovial fluid. The elastic properties of synovial fluid are important in the attenuation of sudden loads to joints, for example, when running.

The formation of hyaluronan molecules within the synovial fluid is dynamic. The orientation of these molecules gives rise to various pores within their configurations. These pores play an important role in the movement of molecules within the synovial fluid. Smaller nutritional molecules move unimpeded (Fig. 13.3A) whereas larger molecules such as inflammatory proteins may become trapped by the hyaluronan meshwork (Fig. 13.3B).

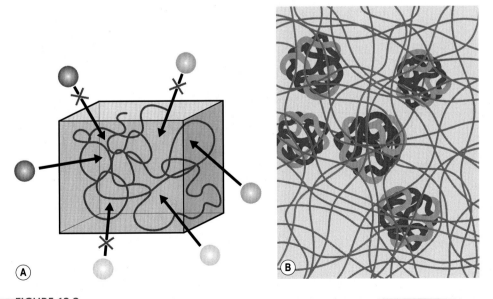

(A) (B)

FIGURE 13.3
Filtration role of HA within synovial fluid. Smaller nutritional molecules move unimpeded (A) whereas larger molecules such as inflammatory proteins may become trapped by the hyaluronan meshwork (B). (From TRB Chemedica [UK] Ltd with permission.)

The hyaluronan in association with joint surface proteins also forms a coating over the entire surface of the joint and plays a further important role in the protection of articular cartilage providing both a barrier to inflammatory mediators and a mechanical lubricating function (Figs 13.4 and 13.5).

FIGURE 13.4
HA forming protective layer over synovium. (From TRB Chemedica [UK] Ltd with permission.)

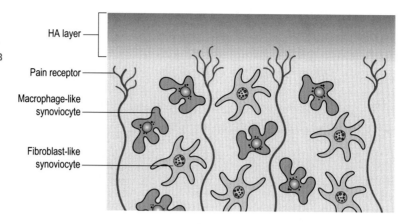

FIGURE 13.5
HA forming protective layer over cartilage. (From TRB Chemedica [UK] Ltd with permission.)

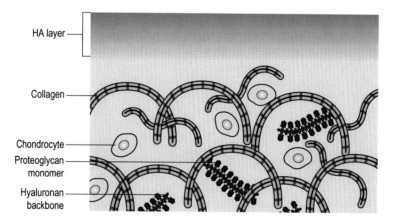

Hyaline cartilage covers the surface of all diarthroidial joints and offers near frictionless contact surfaces at the joint interface. Hyaline cartilage is composed of a small number (as a percentage of cartilage mass) of chondrocytes within a matrix. This extracellular matrix consists of a dense matrix of collagen fibrils and hyaluronan aggregates (hyaluronan and proteoglycans). These aggregates exert a significant osmotic pull causing the cartilage tissue to swell. This hydrophilic property confers a significant amount of the mechanical properties to the articular cartilage.

RATIONALE FOR HA THERAPY IN OSTEOARTHRITIS

Osteoarthritis is characterized by cartilage fibrillation, cartilage loss, subchondral sclerosis, and subchondral bone remodelling. It is now widely accepted however that this degenerative process is underpinned by chronic joint synovitis. Synovial fluid extracted from osteoarthritic joints has been shown to contain raised levels of inflammatory mediators. Further evidence comes from biopsy of affected joints, which demonstrate changes not dissimilar to those seen in rheumatoid arthritis, albeit to a lesser intensity. The presence of various proinflammatory mediators, cytokines, free radicals, and proteinases in the synovial tissue of osteoarthritic joints is believed to adversely influence the function of B fibroblasts, which line the synovial membrane. This in turn results in an altered production of endogenous HA within the joint (Fig. 13.6). The presence of inflammatory mediators has been shown to cause degradation of normal HA within the joint itself.

FIGURE 13.6
The impact of osteoarthritis on normal HA function. (From TRB Chemedica [UK] Ltd with permission.)

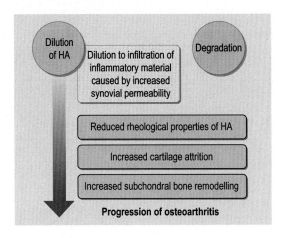

CONCEPT OF VISCOSUPPLEMENTATION

Balazs and Delinger (1993) were the first to describe the concept of "viscosupplementation." Their rationale was to remove the abnormal synovial fluid and replace it with purified high-molecular-weight (MW) HA thereby improving the synovial fluid viscoelasticity. It was believed that this in turn would promote better joint function and thus reduce patient symptoms. Subsequent clinical studies have supported the therapeutic benefits of this technique though two interesting observations arose:

- Therapeutic effects were achieved with lower MW HA than is found in normal synovial fluid
- Clinical effects outlasted the catabolism and known clearance rate of exogenously introduced HA.

These observations suggest that the longer-term clinical benefits observed may involve some other mechanisms and cannot be solely attributed to the immediate mechanical effects following the introduction of a viscoelastic supplement into the joint.

Over 40 studies have been conducted with HA in osteoarthritis of the knee (the most studied joint), but less than a quarter of these represent randomized controlled trials. The majority of these trials compared treatment with placebo in small groups of patients for short periods of time (George 1998).

PHARMACOLOGICAL BASIS OF HA THERAPY

Hyaluronic acid molecules have been shown to bind to specific receptors (CD44 and RHAMM) that are present on the surface membranes of a wide range of cells including those implicated in the pathogenesis of osteoarthritis (inflammatory cells, synoviocytes, chondrocytes). Hyaluronic acid molecules have also been shown to interact with a variety of proteins (hyaladherins) including link proteins in cartilage and those within the pericellular matrix around chondrocytes. As a consequence of the HA interaction with these receptors a variety of intracellular events can be triggered leading to a range of cellular responses (Fig. 13.7).

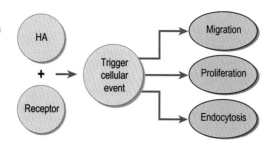

FIGURE 13.7
Triggering of cellular function by HA binding. (From TRB Chemedica [UK] Ltd with permission.)

IS THE MOLECULAR WEIGHT OF EXOGENOUS HA IMPORTANT?

The outcome of HA interaction with its cellular receptors varies subject to a range of local factors (Table 13.1). A major determinant of cellular activity as a result of HA/receptor binding is the size of the HA molecule: the therapeutic window lies between 1 million and around 2.5 million Daltons. The mechanisms that underpin these varied cellular responses remain poorly understood though one explanation suggests that normal interaction between HA molecule and cell involves interaction of a single HA molecule with multiple receptors. Variation in HA molecule size therefore may determine a particular "pattern" of receptor binding determined by HA molecule size.

Table 13.1 Experimental evidence for effect of HA on cellular function

AUTHOR	FINDINGS
Forrester & Wilkinson 1981	The authors investigated the effects of hyaluronate on rabbit neutrophils. They demonstrated that HA at a concentration of 0.7×10^6 Da inhibited leukocyte migration and chemotaxis in a concentration-dependent manner
Takahashi et al. 2000	This study evaluated the effect of intra-articular injections of HA on chondrocyte apoptosis and nitric oxide production using an experimental osteoarthritis model (NZ white rabbits). They demonstrated that HA protects against chondrocyte apoptosis during the development of osteoarthritis, and as such HA may have a valuable chondro-protective effect
Pisko et al. 1983	The authors demonstrated that HA at normal concentrations in joints inhibited polymorphonuclear leukocyte function
Tobetto et al. 1992	The authors investigated the effects of hyaluronan on neutrophil-mediated cartilage. Their results suggested that hyaluronan with a high molecular weight plays an important role in protecting the articular cartilage in inflamed joints from neutrophil injury
Yasuda 2007	The author demonstrated that exogenous HA injected into arthritic joints could act as an inhibitor of proinflammatory cytokines

Although there is good scientific evidence to confirm that MW is an important determinant of biological function of HA, this has been the focus of limited clinical interest and most HA therapy still utilizes HAs with high MWs in the belief that these better fulfill the demands of viscosupplementation as described by Balazs & Delinger (1993). The impact of MW on HAs used therapeutically has yet to be fully elucidated and presents the scientific community with many difficulties due not least to the methodological complexities necessary to investigate this.

COMMON QUESTIONS ABOUT HA THERAPY FROM PATIENTS

Many patients will wish to know why they have been advised to consider a course of HA joint injections and it is important that they understand that the purpose of the injection is to relieve pain and improve function. Patients should however understand that HA injections cannot "undo" cartilage damage as such and that the relief of symptoms may be temporary. Unlike injection of cortisone where significant side effects can develop, HA therapy has been associated with very few complications and may be repeated at appropriate intervals if symptoms return.

Whilst HA therapy results in alterations in a range of complex cellular processes, from the patient's perspective they simply need to know that the purpose of the injection is to restore the normal balance of hyaluronic acid within the joint with the aim of reducing pain and improving function. Modern preparations are prepared by a process of bacterial fermentation and do not contain animal products. As such the risk of allergic reaction is very low. A summary of different HA products is given in Table 13.2.

Table 13.2 Summary of different HA products

PARAMETER	HYALGAN	SYNVISC	OSTENIL – LARGE JOINTS	OSTENIL MINI – SMALL JOINTS
Website	http://www.hyalgan.com	http://www.wyeth.com	http://www.trbchemedica.co.uk	
Source	Rooster combs	Rooster combs	Bacterial fermentation	
License	Knee	Knee	All joints	
Dose	20 mg/2 mL	20 mg/2 mL	20 mg/2 mL	10 mg/1 mL
Number of injections	3–5	3	3–5	3
Allergic reaction	Possible (avian source)	Possible (avian source)	Rare	
Post injection soreness	Uncommon	Uncommon	Rare	

CONTRAINDICATIONS TO HA THERAPY

There are very few absolute contraindications to the use of HA therapy, especially where the HA is that derived from biofermentation as opposed to avian sources, where the risk of allergic reaction is greater. Specific contraindications are given below:

Contraindications to HA Therapy

Contraindications

- Infection in joint
- Systemic infection
- Known allergy

Cautions

- Severe OA changes
- Anticoagulant therapy
- Allergy to bird feathers

SEVERITY OF OSTEOARTHRITIS AND HA THERAPY

The severity of osteoarthritis will influence the therapeutic potential of HA therapy and it is important to remember that this treatment is not the panacea for all arthritic joints. Careful patient evaluation is necessary involving both clinical and usually radiographic assessment before deciding to embark on this line of treatment. A key indicator of success is the degree of osteoarthritic change within the joint and this does not necessarily correlate well with the level of reported symptoms. Whilst there are many grading scales put forward describing and quantifying pathological changes in joints, Kellgren & Lawrence (1957) provide a simple four-point scale that incorporates the amount of local osteophytosis (Fig. 13.8). This is particularly important as osteophytosis can often be quite marked when dealing with the lower limb and is a major cause of pain and functional disturbance. Where osteophytosis is marked HA therapy may not prove optimal as much of the joint pain is mediated by mechanical impingement of the joint. An example of early osteoarthritis of the 1st metatarsophalangeal joint that responded well to HA therapy is given in Fig. 13.9.

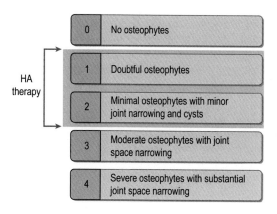

HA therapy	0	No osteophytes
	1	Doubtful osteophytes
	2	Minimal osteophytes with minor joint narrowing and cysts
	3	Moderate osteophytes with joint space narrowing
	4	Severe osteophytes with substantial joint space narrowing

FIGURE 13.8
Kellgren & Lawrence Scale (1957) and role of HA therapy. (From TRB Chemedica [UK] Ltd with permission.)

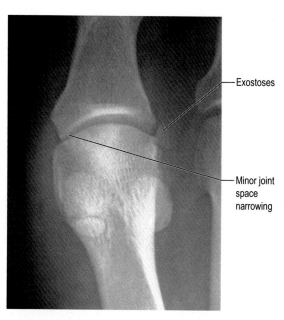

Exostoses

Minor joint space narrowing

FIGURE 13.9
Early osteoarthritis of the 1st metatarsophalangeal joint that responded well to HA therapy.

INJECTION TECHNIQUE

Even though the risks of complications are very low, informed consent is required prior to the administration of any joint injection. This should include a full explanation of the rationale of treatment and risks and benefits of HA therapy together with details of alternative treatment strategies. Best practice suggests that this consent is obtained in writing but remember that consent can be written without being informed.

All joint injections should be given after thorough antiseptic skin prep and strict aseptic precautions. Most if not all HAs come in preloaded syringes but if they have to be drawn up a fresh sterile needle should be used to further minimize the risk of cross-infection. The techniques are the same as described in Chapter 11.

TIME LINE OF THERAPEUTIC EFFECTS

HA therapy frequently does not produce immediate clinical improvement and this is certainly the case for treatment of larger joints such as the knee and ankle. Smaller joints may show a more rapid clinical response. Injections are repeated at weekly intervals subject to there being no adverse reactions. It is usual to see a cumulative response over this time period with continued clinical benefit beyond the period of the last injection.

REPEATING TREATMENT

Subject to appropriate clinical reassessment HA therapy may be repeated in accordance with the patient's symptoms. The authors' preference for a first metatarsophalangeal joint is three weekly injections of Ostenil mini. Practically one should consider the appropriateness of continued courses of HA therapy once the interval of relief of symptoms drops below 6 months.

PROLOTHERAPY

INTRODUCTION

Prolotherapy is a technique often employed to treat tendon injuries. Injection of "proliferating agents" into injured tendons and ligaments is claimed to stimulate the body's natural healing mechanisms thereby leading to the resolution/repair of previously injured tissues. The term "proliferating agent" refers to a substance which when injected into an area of injured tissue acts as an irritant, stimulating various components of the body's own healing response. There are three principal types of proliferating agents:

- Irritants – These were the first class of proliferants used by prolotherapists. They include phenol, guaiacol and tannic acid. Each of these compounds leads to either direct cellular injury or results in the cells becoming antigenic. The end result is that they evoke an inflammatory response at the site of injection.
- Osmotics – These act by dehydrating cells at the injection site by osmosis. Injection of concentrated glucose solution leads to disruption of the normal cellular osmotic concentrations; intracellular fluid is lost and cell death occurs. The net result is the same as with injection of irritants in that a local inflammatory response is evoked.

- Chemotactics – Sodium morrhuate is the sodium salt of the fatty acid component derived from cod liver oil. Fish oils are rich in polyunsaturated fatty acids, such as arachidonic acid. Arachidonic acid is a direct biosynthetic precursor to inflammatory mediators such as prostaglandins and leukotrienes. Injection of sodium morrhuate has been shown to lead to a local inflammatory response.

A selected bibliography for prolotherapy references appears at the end of the chapter.

MECHANISM OF ACTION

Prolotherapy has been utilized for a range of conditions since the late 1950s with the first medical publications appearing in the very early 1960s. Despite this history, prolotherapy has only recently found increased acceptance within the medical community. Applications are broad, ranging from the management of cervical instability to treatment of chronic back pain and sciatica.

The mechanism by which this therapy is believed to work is not well defined though a number of theories have been postulated. One theory is based on our current understanding of the normal wound healing processes. We know that as a result of local injury chemotactic factors are released leading to the influx of granulocytes to the area of injury. These cells play an important role in the phagocytosis of cellular debris as well as attracting other cell types essential to the wound healing process (monocytes and macrophages). This initial phase of inflammation, which lasts 2–3 days, is followed by a late inflammatory phase lasting 7–10 days. During this period monocytes and macrophages play a vital role in clearing cellular debris and pathogens. Throughout the early and late inflammatory phases chemotactic factors for fibroblasts are released.

Fibroblasts are stimulated to produce new intercellular matrix, including new collagen essential for the tissue repair process. The early granulation tissue laid down by fibroblasts also contains large numbers of granulocytes and macrophages within a mix of intercellular matrix and collagen. Ultimately as the process of removing cellular debris is completed and granulocytes die these are removed by macrophages, which in turn migrate away from the injury site. Fibroblasts remain and continue the process of repair and remodelling of the injured tissue, a process that lasts for several months. As the injured tissue remodels the new collagen undergoes structural alterations, strengthening and contracting. It is this latter process that is believed to be critical to the theoretical basis of prolotherapy.

Advocates of prolotherapy believe that injection of an irritant into injured ligament evokes an acute inflammatory response and ultimately the deposition of new collagen by fibroblasts. Following maturation of the repair process the newly deposited collagen is remodelled leading to contracture and thus strengthening the ligament.

GROWTH FACTORS

Growth factors may represent a new direction for the treatment of soft tissue injuries. These may, subject to appropriate clinical evidence and licensing, become incorporated into the field of prolotherapy. Growth factors have been developed and applied to stimulate the repair of various cells, organs, and diseases. Polypeptide growth factors act directly upon fibroblasts (which make collagen). Epidermal growth factor, insulin-like growth factors, fibroblast growth factors, and platelet-derived growth factors are now available for research and testing purposes.

SCLEROSING INJECTIONS

CHEMICAL NEUROLYSIS OF MORTON'S NEUROMA

Dockery has published a number of papers on the use of sclerosing injections in the treatment of intermetatarsal (Morton's) neuromas. He credits the technique to Dr. MD Steinberg who he first heard lecture on the subject of dilute alcohol injections and vitamin B12 injections for neuromas in 1973 (Dockery 2002). Ethanol produces neuritis and Wallerian nerve degeneration or chemical neurolysis when absorbed into nerve tissue. Dockery postulates that repeated injections of this dilute solution in close proximity to nerve tissue causes selective degeneration or neurolysis until the nerve completely ceases to function or is directly destroyed.

Dockery published his technique for mixing the solution in 1986 and the different clinical conditions responsive to sclerosing injections. He evaluated more than 150 patients who underwent weekly injections of 0.5 mL of a 4% alcohol solution for clinical symptoms of intermetatarsal neuromas. The results showed that more than 80% of patients experienced resolution of their neuroma symptoms after three or more weekly injections (Dockery & Nilson 1986). The mixture was initially composed of 48 mL of 2% lidocaine with epinephrine (1:100 000) and 2 mL of ethanol (dehydrated ethyl alcohol), which resulted in a 4% dilute solution. Further research led to the development of mixing 48 mL of 0.5% bupivacaine HCl with epinephrine (1:200 000) with 2 mL of dehydrated ethyl alcohol for injection, for a total volume of 50 mL (Dockery 1999). Of the 100 patients included in Dockery's 1999 study, 73 females and 27 males received injections of a 4% solution. Follow-up evaluation was performed for each patient at 6 months to 2 years (average 13 months) following completion of treatment. His results showed that 82 patients reported 100% improvement of their symptoms and seven patients reported from 60% to 85% improvement. This resulted in an overall patient satisfaction rate of excellent or good of 89%. Eleven patients had continued pain or other symptoms at the end of the study and elected to proceed with surgical neurectomy. This paper prompted one of the authors (Reilly) to utilize alcohol therapy for intermetatarsal neuromas following a failure of surgical management, in an unpublished study at the Northampton School of Podiatry (2001).

Other authors (Fanucci et al. 2004; Hyer et al. 2005; Hughes et al. 2007) have gone on to use alcohol solutions at various strengths, notably Hughes et al. (2007) who reported on their results of a 20% alcohol injection under sonographic guidance.

FILLERS

Physiological filling materials such as dermis, fascia, and fat have been used as autologous implants for tissue augmentation for many years, with specific surgical techniques used for each substance (Gampper et al. 2007). A range of injectable filling materials including collagen, HA cutting oils, paraffin, and silicone is now available.

The ideal filling material has the following qualities:

- Physiological – it should incorporate itself with the body's tissues
- Simple procedure – easy to inject
- Risk free – there should be no complications or adverse effects
- Permanent – it should not degrade with time.

Gampper et al. (2007) state that the depth of the defect should determine the filler chosen for the appropriate procedure:

- Superficial defects – collagen, hyaluronic acid polymers
- Deeper defects – fat, synthetic materials, silicone, implants, or permanent fillers.

Collagen fillers can be divided into those of bovine and human origin, with bovine products such as Zyderm being the most widely employed. Restylane and Perlane are composed of hyaluronic acid, both derived from bacteria that produce hyaluronic acid. In cosmetic surgery, Restylane is used for superficial wrinkles, while Perlane, which is much less susceptible to breakdown in the body, is used for deeper wrinkles. They can be used as plantar fat pad replacement: results can last as long as 1 year. Sculptra is composed of poly-L-lactic acid. This material has been used for years to make suture materials and is known to be highly biocompatible.

Silicone or polymerized siloxanes are mixed inorganic–organic polymers. Silicones can be synthesized with a wide variety of properties and compositions. They vary in consistency from liquid to gel and rubber to hard plastic (Wu 2008). The physical properties of silicone make it an ideal biomaterial. It is chemically inert, noncarcinogenic, capable of sterilization, not physically modified by soft tissue, noninflammatory, capable of resisting mechanical strains, and produces no state of allergy or hypersensitivity.

Injected liquid silicone (ILS) has been used for decades with a high level of reported success and minimal side effects (Balkin 1966, 1975, 1977, 1984, 2005; Balkin and Kaplin 1991). Nearly a decade ago, van Schie and coworkers reported on the results of a randomized clinical trial that strongly corroborated past anecdotal reports, suggesting that peak plantar pressures could be reduced and plantar tissue thickness increased through the use of ILS in areas of high plantar pressure and callus/lesions (Van Schie et al. 2002). Medical fluid silicone products, such as Innopad, appear to be safe, effective, and stable biomaterial for treating weight-bearing loss of plantar fat and other high-pressure points.

BOTULINUM TOXIN

Vlahovic et al. (2008) reported a 3-month follow-up of two patients who received injections of botulinum toxin type A (Botox, Allergan Inc, Irvine, CA), a purified neurotoxin complex, for hyperhidrosis. Both patients received intradermal injections of Botox into the plantar aspect of both feet. The authors found it to be an effective and safe treatment for plantar hyperhidrosis.

Radovic & Shah (2008) reported the use of botulinum toxin A injection to reduce a hallux abducto valgus deformity clinically and radiographically and also its associated pain.

REFERENCES

Balazs, E.A., Delinger, J.L., 1993. Viscosupplementation: a new concept in the treatment of osteoarthritis. J. Rheumatol. 39 (Suppl.), 3–9.

Balkin, S.W., 1966. Silicone injection for plantar keratoses: preliminary report. J. Am. Podiatry Assoc. 56, 1–11.

Balkin, S.W., 1975. Treatment of corns by injectable silicone. Arch. Dermatol. 111, 1143–1145.

Balkin, S.W., 1977. Treatment of painful scars on soles and digits with injections of fluid silicone. J. Dermatol. Surg. Oncol. 3 (6), 612–614.

Balkin, S.W., 1984. The fluid silicone prosthesis. Clin. Podiatry 1 (1), 145–164.

Balkin, S.W., 2005. Injectable silicone and the foot: a 41-year clinical and histologic history. Dermatol. Surg. 31, 1555–1559; discussion 1560.

Balkin, S.W., Kaplan, L., 1991. Silicone injection management of diabetic foot ulcers: a possible model for prevention of pressure ulcers. Decubitus 4 (4), 38–40.

Dockery, G.L., 1999. The treatment of intermetatarsal neuromas with 4% alcohol sclerosing injections. J. Foot Ankle Surg. 38, 403–406.

Dockery, G.L., 2002. Is injection therapy the best solution for foot neuromas? Podiatry Today 15, 22–25.

Dockery, G.L., Nilson, R.Z., 1986. Intralesional injections. Clin. Podiatr. Med. Surg. 3, 473–485.

Fanucci, E., Masala, S., Fabiano, S., et al., 2004. Treatment of intermetatarsal Morton's neuroma with alcohol injection under US guide: 10-month follow up. Eur. Radiol. 14 (3), 514–518.

Forrester, J.V., Wilkinson, P.C., 1981. Inhibition of leukocyte locomotion by hyaluronic acid. J. Cell. Sci. 48, 315–331.

Gampper, T.J., Tholpady, A., Monheit, G.D., Kayal, J.D., 2007. Collagen Injections. Available at: http://emedicine.medscape.com/article/1271282-overview (updated: May 3 2007).

George, E., 1998. Intra-articular hyaluronan treatment for osteoarthritis. Ann. Rheum. Dis. 57, 637–640.

Hughes, R.J., Ali, K., Jones, H., Kendall, S., Connell, D.A., 2007. Treatment of Morton's neuroma with alcohol injection under sonographic guidance: follow-up of 101 cases. AJR 188, 1535–1539.

Hyer, C.F., Mehl, L.R., Block, A.J., Vancourt, R.B., 2005. Treatment of recalcitrant intermetatarsal neuroma with 4% sclerosing alcohol injection: a pilot study. J. Foot Ankle Surg. 44, 287–291.

Kellgren, J.H., Lawrence, J.S., 1957. Radiological assessment of osteo-arthrosis. Ann. Rheum. Dis. 16 (4), 494–502.

Pisko, E.J., Turner, R.A., Soderstrom, L.P., et al., 1983. Inhibition of neutrophil phagocytosis and enzyme release by hyaluronic acid. Clin. Exp. Rheumatol. 1, 41–44.

Radovic, P.A., Shah, E., 2008. Nonsurgical treatment for hallux abducto valgus with botulinum toxin A. J. Am. Podiatr. Med. Assoc. 98, 61–65.

Takahashi, K., Hashimoto, S., Kubo, T., et al., 2000. Effect of hyaluronan on chondrocyte apoptosis and nitric oxide production in experimentally induced osteoarthritis. J. Rheumatol. 27, 1713–1720.

Tobetto, K., Yasui, T., Ando, T., 1992. Inhibition effect of hyaluronan on 14C arachidonic acid release from labeled human synovial fibroblasts. Jpn. J. Pharmacol. 60, 79–84.

van Schie, C.H., Whalley, A., Armstrong, D.G., Vileikyte, L., Boulton, A.J., 2002. The effect of silicone injections in the diabetic foot on peak plantar pressure and plantar tissue thickness: a 2-year follow-up. Arch. Phys. Med. Rehab. 83, 919–923.

Vlahovic, T.C., Dunn, P.S., Blau, J.C., Gauthier, C., 2008. Injectable botulinum toxin as a treatment for plantar hyperhidrosis: a case study. J. Am. Podiatr. Med. Assoc. 98, 156–159.

Wu, S.C., 2008. Injectable silicone: can it mitigate plantar pedal pressure? Podiatry Today 21 (9).

Yasuda, T., 2007. Hyaluronan inhibits cytokine production by lipopolysaccharide-stimulated U937 macrophages through down-regulation of NF-B via ICAM-1. Inflamm. Res. 56 (6), 246–253.

BIBLIOGRAPHY AND FURTHER READING

Altman, R.D., Moskowitz, R., 1998. Intra-articular sodium hyaluronate (HyalganÒ) in the treatment of patients with osteoarthritis of the knee: a randomized clinical trial. J. Rheumatol. 25, 2203–2212.

Balazs, E.A., Watson, D., Duff, I.F., Roseman, S., 1967. Hyaluronic acid in synovial fluid. I. Molecular parameters of hyaluronic acid in normal and arthritic fluids. Arthritis Rheum. 10, 357–376.

Bragatini, A., Cassini, M., DeBastiani, G., Perbellini, A., 1987. Controlled single blind trial of intra-articularly injected hyaluronic acid (hyalgan) in osteoarthritis of the knee. Clin. Trials J. 24, 333–340.

Carpenter, B., Motley, T., 2008. The role of viscosupplementation in the ankle using hylan G-F 20. J. Foot Ankle Surg. 47, 377–384.

Centeno, C.J., et al., 2005. Fluoroscopically guided cervical prolotherapy for instability with blinded pre and post radiographic reading. Pain Physician 8, 67–72.

Chasan, P.E., 2007. The history of injectable silicone fluids for soft-tissue augmentation. Plast. Reconstr. Surg. 120 (7), 2034–2040; discussion 2041–2033.

Dagenai, S., Haldeman s, J.R., 2005. Intraligamentous injection of sclerosing solutions (prolotherapy) for spinal pain: a critical review of the literature. Spine J. 5, 310–328.

Dahl, L.B., Dahl, I.M.S., Engstrom-Laurent, A., Granath, K., 1985. Concentration and molecular weight of sodium hyaluronate in synovial fluid from patients with rheumatoid arthritis and other arthropathies. Ann. Rheum. Dis. 44, 817–822.

Dixon, AStJ., Jacoby, R.K., Berry, H., et al., 1988. Clinical trial of sodium hyaluronate in patients with osteoarthritis of the knee. Curr. Med. Opin. 11, 205–213.

Forrester, J.V., Lackie, J.M., 1981. Effect of hyaluronic acid on neutrophil adhesion. J. Cell Sci. 50, 329–344.

Jubb, R., Piva, S., Beinat, L., Dacre, J., Gishen, P., 2001. Structure modification in osteoarthritis with intra-articular sodium hyaluronate of mol. 500–730 kDa. Ann. Rheum. Dis. 60 (Suppl. 1), 46.

Kayfetz, D.O., 1963. Occipito-cervical (whiplash) injuries treated with prolotherapy. Med. Trial Tech. Q. 9, 9–29 passim.

Kayfetz, D.O., et al., 1963. Whiplash injury and other ligamentous headache – its management with prolotherapy. Headache 3, 21–28.

Kopp, S., Carlsson, G.E., Haraldson, T., Wenneberg, B., 1987. Long term effect of intra-articular injections of sodium hyaluronate and corticosteroid on temperomandibular joint arthritis. J. Oral Maxillofac Surg. 45, 929–935.

Maxwell, N.J., Ryan, M.B., Taunton, J.E., Gillies, J.H., Wong, A.D., 2007. Sonographically guided intratendinous injection of hyperosmolar dextrose to treat chronic tendinosis of the Achilles tendon: a pilot study. AJR 189, W215–W220.

Merriman, J.R., 1964. Prolotherapy versus operative fusion in the treatment of joint instability of the spine and pelvis. J. Int. Coll. Surg. 42, 150–159.

Mozena, J.D., Clifford, J.T., 2007. Efficacy of chemical neurolysis for the treatment of interdigital nerve compression of the foot: a retrospective study. J. Am. Podiatr. Med. Assoc. 97, 203–206.

Mulder, G.D., Jahnigen, D., Vandepol, C.J., 1988. The role of injectable collagen in the prevention of recurrent diabetic ulcers. J. Am. Podiatr. Med. Assoc. 78, 238–242.

Munteanu, S.E., Menz, H.B., Zammit, G.V., et al., 2009. Efficacy of intra-articular hyaluronan (Synvisc) for the treatment of osteoarthritis affecting the first metatarsophalangeal joint of the foot (hallux limitus): study protocol for a randomized placebo controlled trial. J. Foot Ankle Res. doi:10.1186/1757-1146-2-2.

Namiki, O., Toyoshima, H., Morisaki, N., 1982. Therapeutic effect of intra-articular injection of high molecular weight hyaluronic acid on osteoarthritis of the knee. Int. J. Clin. Pharmacol. Toxicol. 20, 501–507.

Narins, R.S., Beer, K., 2006. Liquid injectable silicone: a review of its history, immunology, technical considerations, complications, and potential. Plast. Reconstr. Surg. 118 (Suppl. 3), 77S–84S.

Peyron, J.G., Balazs, E.A., 1974. Preliminary clinical assessment of Na hyaluronate injection into human arthritic joints. Pathol. Biol. 22, 731–736.

Pons, M., Alvarez, F., Solana, R., 2007. Sodium hyaluronate in the treatment of hallux rigidus. a single-blind, randomized study. Foot Ankle Int. 28 (1), 38–42.

Prather, C.L., Jones, D.H., 2006. Liquid injectable silicone for soft tissue augmentation. Dermatol. Ther. 19 (3), 159–168.

Price, R.D., Berry, M.G., Navsaria, H.A., 2007. Hyaluronic acid: the scientific and clinical evidence. J. Plast. Reconstr. Aesth. Surg. 60, 1110–1119.

Punzi, L., Schiavon, F., Ramonda, R., et al., 1988. Intra articular hyaluronic acid in the treatment of inflammatory and non-inflammatory knee effusions. Curr. Therep. Res. 43, 643–647.

Schichikawa, K., Maeda, A., Ogawa, N., 1983. Clinical studies of the intra-articular injection of sodium hyaluronate in the treatment of osteoarthritis of human knee. Ryumachi 23, 280–290.

Schichikawa, K., Maeda, A., Ogawa, N., 1983. Evaluation of drug effectiveness of sodium hyaluronate for osteoarthritis deformans of the knee. Rheumatism 23, 280–290.

Smith, M.M., Ghosh, P., 1987. The synthesis of hyaluronic acid by human synovial fibroblasts is influenced by the nature of the hyaluronate in the extracellular environment. Rheumatol. Int. 7, 113–122.

Wu, S.C.S., Bevilacqua, N.J., Rogers, L.C., Armstrong, D.G., 2006. Tissue volumizing: can we create an internal orthotic? Podiatry Today 19 (10).

Yamamoto, R., Namiki, O., Iwata, H., et al., 1988. Dose finding test of SPH (high molecular weight sodium hyaluronate) in patients with periarthritis scapulohemeralis. J. Clin. Therap. Med. 2102–2120.

Yamamoto, R., Namiki, O., Iwata, H., et al., 1988. Randomized comparative study of sodium hyaluronate (SPH) on periarthritis scapulohemeralis. Jap. J. Clin. Pharmacol. Ther. 19, 717–733.

Zappi, E., Barnett, J.G., Zappi, M., Barnett, C.R., 2007. The long-term host response to liquid silicone injected during soft tissue augmentation procedures: a microscopic appraisal. Dermatol. Surg. 33 (Suppl. 2), S186–S192; discussion S192.

SUBJECT INDEX

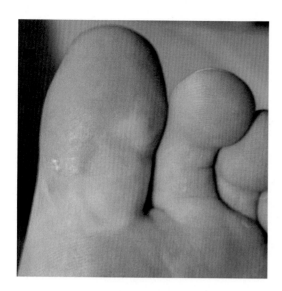

PLATE-1
Hallux block sequence step 3.

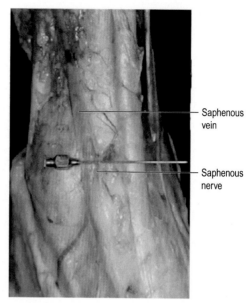

Saphenous
vein

Saphenous
nerve

PLATE-2
Saphenous nerve.

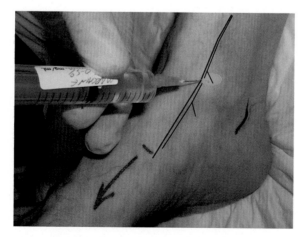

PLATE-3
Saphenous block injection technique.

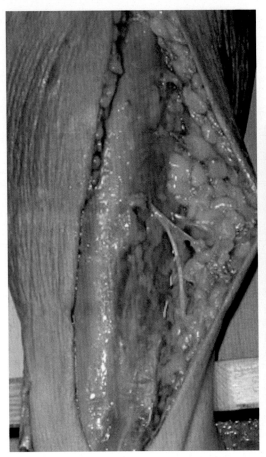

PLATE-4
Superficial fibular nerve.

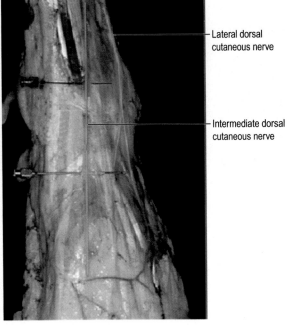

Lateral dorsal cutaneous nerve

Intermediate dorsal cutaneous nerve

PLATE-5
Superficial fibular nerve at the ankle.

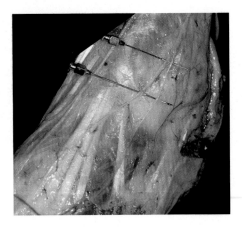

PLATE-6
Superficial fibular (peroneal) nerve.

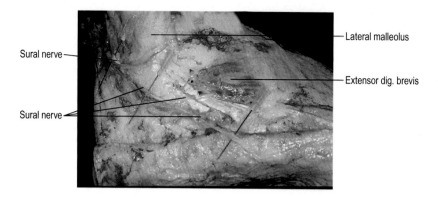

Sural nerve —

Sural nerve ◄—

Lateral malleolus

Extensor dig. brevis

PLATE-7
Sural nerve.

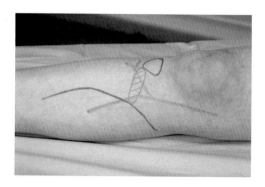

PLATE-8
Saphenous nerve block (knee) technique.

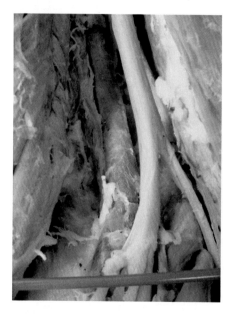

PLATE-9
Rear dissection of right popliteal fossa
showing popliteal nerve branching.

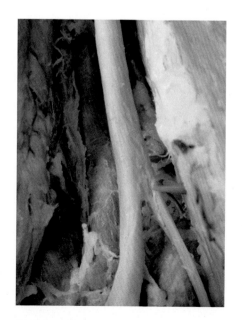

PLATE-10
Danger zone of inappropriate needle placement.

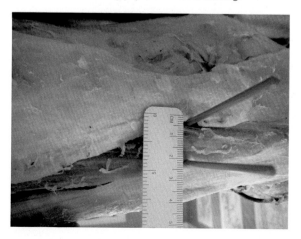

PLATE-11
Danger zone of inappropriate needle placement.

ELSEVIER DVD-ROM LICENCE AGREEMENT

Printed in the United States
By Bookmasters